D0045585

DISCARD

DISCARD

THE CEREBRAL CODE

Books by WILLIAM H. CALVIN

The Cerebral Code
How Brains Think
*Conversations with Neil's Brain**
How the Shaman Stole the Moon
The Ascent of Mind
The Cerebral Symphony
The River That Flows Uphill
The Throwing Madonna
*Inside the Brain**

*with GEORGE A. OJEMANN

THE CEREBRAL CODE

Thinking a Thought in the Mosaics of the Mind

WILLIAM H. CALVIN

A Bradford Book
The MIT Press
Cambridge, Massachusetts
London, England

Copyright ©1996 by William H. Calvin
   All rights reserved.   Except for brief excerpts and personal
   photocopying of a single chapter, no part of this book may be
   reproduced in any form (including information storage and retrieval,
   photocopying, and recording) without permission from the
   publisher.

WCalvin@U.Washington.edu
http://weber.u.washington.edu/~wcalvin/

Supplements and corrections to this book can be found on the web
page *http://weber.u.washington.edu/~wcalvin/bk9.html*

This book was designed, and set in Palatino, by the author;
it was printed and bound in the USA.

                        Printing history
    10   9   8   7   6   5   4   3   2   1   96   97   98   99   2000   01

            Library of Congress Cataloging-in-Publication Data

Calvin, William H., 1939-
   The cerebral code : thinking a thought in the mosaics of the mind /
   William H. Calvin.
      p. cm.
   "A Bradford book."
   Includes bibliographical references and index.
   ISBN: 0-262-03241-4 (alk. paper)
   1. Cognitive neuroscience. 2. Thought and thinking. 3. Cerebral
cortex. 4. Natural selection. I. Title.
   [DNLM: 1. Memory -- physiology. 2. Thinking -- physiology. 3.
Brain -- physiology. 4. Consciousness -- physiology.
WL 102 C168c 1996]
QL360.5.C35 1996
612.8'2--dc20
DNLM/DLC for Library of Congress   96-17644

Contents

Prologue

There may be nothing new under the sun, but
permutation of the old within complex systems
can do wonders.

STEPHEN JAY GOULD, 1977

THIS IS A BOOK about thought, memory, creativity, consciousness, narrative, talking to oneself, and even dreaming. In
a book that parallels this one, *How Brains Think*, I explored
those subjects in a general way but here I treat them as some of the
predicted outcomes of a detailed darwinian theory for how our
cerebral cortex represents mental images — and occasionally
recombines them, to create something new and different.

This book proposes how darwinian processes could operate in
the brain to shape up mental images. Starting with shuffled
memories no better than the jumble of our nighttime dreams, a
mental image can evolve into something of quality, such as a
sentence to speak aloud. Jung said that dreaming goes on continuously but you can't see it when you are awake, just as you can't
see the stars in the daylight because the sky is too bright. Mine is
a theory for what goes on, hidden from view by the glare of
waking mental operations, that produces our peculiarly human
type of consciousness with its versatile intelligence. As Piaget
emphasized, intelligence is what we use when we don't know
what to do, when we have to grope rather than using a standard
response. In this book, I tackle a mechanism for doing this
exploration and improvement offline, how we think before we act
and how we practice the art of good guessing.

Surprisingly, the subtitle's *mosaics of the mind* is not just a literary metaphor. It is a description of mechanism at what appears to be an appropriate level of explanation for many mental phenomena — that of hexagonal mosaics of electrical activity, competing for territory in the association cortex of the brain. This two-dimensional mosaic is predicted to grow and dissolve, much as the sugar crystals do in the bottom of a supersaturated glass of iced tea. Looking down on the cortical surface, with the right kind of imaging, ought to reveal a constantly changing patchwork quilt.

A closer look at each patch ought to reveal a hexagonal pattern that repeats every 0.5 mm. The pattern within each hexagon of this mosaic may be the representation of an item of our vocabulary: objects and actions such as the cat that sat on the mat, tunes such as Beethoven's dit-dit-dit-dah, images such as the profile of your grandmother, a high-order concept such as a Turing Machine — even something for which you have no word, such as the face of someone whose name you haven't learned. If I am right, the spatiotemporal firing pattern within that hexagon is your cerebral code for a word or mental image.

THE OTHER PHRASE IN THE BOOK'S TITLE that is sure to be mistaken for literary license is, of course, the *cerebral code*. The word "code" is often only a short way of saying "unlocking the secrets of" and newspaper headline writers love such short words. Neurobiologists also speak loosely about codes, as when we talk of "frequency codes" and "place codes," when we really mean only a simple mapping.

Real codes are phrase-based translation tables, such as those of bank wires and diplomatic telegrams. A code is a translation table whereby short abstract phrases are elaborated into the "real thing." It's similar to looking up *ambivalence* in a dictionary and getting an explanatory sentence back. In the genetic code, the RNA nucleotide sequence *CUU* is translated into leucine, the triplet *GGA* into glycine, and so on. The cerebral code, strictly speaking, would be what we use to convert thought into action, a translation table between the short-form cerebral pattern and its muscular implementation.

Informally, *code* is also used for the short-form pattern itself, for instance, a nucleotide chain such as *GCACUUCUUGCACUU*. In this book, *cerebral code* refers to the spatiotemporal firing pattern of neocortical neurons that is essential to represent a concept, word, or image, even a metaphor. One of my theoretical results is that a unique code could be contained within a unit hexagon about 0.5 mm across (though it is often redundantly repeated in many neighboring hexagons).

It was once thought that the genetic code was universal, that all organisms from bacteria to people used the same translation table. Now it turns out that mitochondria use a somewhat different translation table. Although the cerebral code is a true code, it surely isn't going to be universal; I doubt that the spatiotemporal firing pattern I use for *dog* (transposed to a musical scale, it would be a short melody, perhaps with some chords) is the same one that you use. Each person's cerebral codes are probably an accident of development and childhood experience. If we find some commonality, for example, that most people's brains innately use a particular subset of codes for animate objects (say, C minor chords) and another subset (like the D major chords) for inanimate objects, I will be pleasantly surprised.

An important consequence of my cerebral code candidate, falling out of the way in which cortical pattern-copying mechanisms seem capable of generating new categories, is that ascending levels of abstraction become possible — even analogies can compete, to help you answer those multiple-choice questions such as "*A* is to *B* as *C* is to *D,E,F*." With a darwinian process operating in cerebral cortex, you can imagine using stratified stability to generate those strata of concepts that are inexpressible except by roundabout, inadequate means — as when we know things of which we cannot speak. That's the topic of the book's penultimate chapter, "The Making of Metaphor."

AS A NEUROPHYSIOLOGIST with long experience doing single neuron recordings in locales ranging from sea slug ganglia *in vitro* to human cerebral cortex *in situ*, I undertook this theoretical venture about a decade ago. I didn't set out to explain representations, or even the nature of working memory. Like most people in neurobiology, I considered such questions too big to be approached directly. One had to work on their foundations instead.

Back then, I had a much more modest goal: to seek brain analogies to the darwinian mechanisms that create higher-order complex systems in nature, something that could handle Kenneth Craik's 1943 notion of simulating a possible course of action before actually acting. We know, after all, that the darwinian ratchet can create advanced capabilities in stages, that it's an algorithmic process that gradually creates quality — and gets around the usual presumption that fancy things require an even fancier designer. We even know a lot of the ins-and-outs of the process, such as how evolution speeds up in island settings and why it slows down in continental ones.

However attractive a top-down cognitive design process might be, we know that a bottom-up darwinian process can achieve sophisticated results, given enough time. Perhaps the brain has invented something even fancier than darwinism, but we first ought (so I reasoned) to try the darwinian algorithm out for size, as a foundation — and then look for shortcuts. In 1987, I wrote a commentary in *Nature*, "The brain as a Darwin Machine," proposing a term for any full-fledged darwinian process, in analogy to the Turing Machine.

Indeed, since William James first discussed the matter in the 1870s during Charles Darwin's lifetime, darwinian processes have been thought to be a possible basis for mental processes, a way to shape up a grammatically correct sentence or a more efficient plan for visiting the essential aisles of the grocery store. They're a way to explore the Piagetian maze, where you don't initially know what to do; standard neural decision trees for overlearned items may suffice for answering questions, but something creative is often needed when deciding what to do next — as when you pose a question.

When first discovered by Darwin and Wallace and used to explain the shaping up of new species over many millennia, the darwinian ratchet was naturally thought to operate slowly. Then it was discovered that a darwinian shaping up of antibodies also occurs, during the days-to-weeks time course of the immune response to a novel antigen. You end up with a new type of antibody that is a hundred times more effective than the ones available at the time of infection — and is, of course, far more numerous as well. What would it take, one asks, for the brain to mimic this creative mechanism using still faster neural mechanisms to run essentially the same process? Might some milliseconds-to-minutes darwinian ratchet form the foundation, atop which our sophisticated mental life is built?

As Wittgenstein once observed, you gain insights mostly through new arrangements of things you already know, not by acquiring new data. This is certainly true at the level of biological variation: despite the constant talk of "mutations," it's really the random shuffle of grandparent chromosomes during meiosis as sperm and ova are made, and the subsequent sexual recombination during fertilization, that generates the substantial new variations, such as all the differences between siblings. Novel mental images have also been thought to arise from recombinations during brain activity. In our waking hours, most of these surely remain at subconscious levels — but many are probably the same sorts of juxtapositions that we experience in dreams every night. As the neurophysiologist J. Allan Hobson has noted:

> Persons, places, and time change suddenly, without notice. There may be abrupt jumps, cuts, and interpolations. There may be fusions: impossible combinations of people, places, times, and activity abound.

Most such juxtapositions and chimeras are nonsense. But during our waking hours, they might be better shaped up in a darwinian manner. Only the more realistic ones might normally reach "consciousness."

THE MECHANISTIC REQUIREMENTS for this kind of darwinian process are now better known than they were in the 1870s; they go well beyond the selective-survival summary of darwinism that so often trivializes the issue. Charles Darwin, alas, named his theory *natural selection*, thus leading many of his followers to focus on only one of what are really a half-dozen essential aspects of the darwinian process. Thus far, most "darwinian" discussions of the brain's ontogeny, when examined, turn out to involve only several of the darwinian essentials — and not the whole creative loop that I discuss in later chapters.

I attempted to apply these six darwinian attributes to our mental processes in *The Cerebral Symphony* and in "Islands in the mind," published in *Seminars in the Neurosciences* in 1991, but at that time I hadn't yet found a specific neural mechanism that could turn the crank. Later in 1991, I realized that two recent developments in neuroscience — emergent synchrony and standard-length intracortical axons — provided the essential elements needed for a darwinian process to operate in the superficial layers of our cerebral cortex. This neocortical Darwin Machine opens up a broad neurophysiological-level consideration of cortical operation. With it, you can address a range of cognitive issues, from recognition memory to higher intellectual function including language and plan-ahead mechanisms — even figuring out what goes with the leftovers in the refrigerator.

DESPITE THE HERITAGE from William James and Kenneth Craik, despite the recent interdisciplinary enthusiasm for fresh darwinian and complex adaptive systems approaches to long-standing problems, any such darwinian crank is going to seem new to those scientists who have little detailed knowledge of darwinian principles beyond the crude "survival of the fittest" caricature.

For one thing, you have to think about the statistical nature of the forest, as well as the characteristic properties of each type of tree. Population thinking is not an easily acquired habit but I hope that the first chapter will briefly illustrate how to use it to make a list of six essential features of the darwinian process — plus a few more features that serve as catalysts, to turn the ratchet faster. Next comes a dose of the local neural circuits of cerebral cortex, as that is where the triangular arrays of synchronized neurons are predicted, that will be needed for both the coding and creative complexity aspects. This is also where I introduce the hexagon as the smallest unit of the Hebbian cell-assembly and estimate its size as about 100 minicolumns involving 10,000 neurons (it's essentially the 0.5 mm macrocolumn of association cortex, about the same size as the ocular dominance columns of primary visual cortex but perhaps not anchored as permanently). This is where compressing the code is discussed and that puts us in a position to appreciate how long-term memory might work, both for encoding and retrieval.

About halfway through the book, we'll be finished with the circuitry of a neocortical Darwin Machine and ready to consider, in *Act II*, some of its surprising products: categories, cross-modality matching, sequences, analogies, and metaphors. It's just like the familiar distinction we make between the principles of evolution and the products of evolution. The products, in this case, are some of the most interesting ways that humans differ from our ape cousins: going beyond mere category formation to shape up further levels of complexity such as metaphor, narrative, and even agendas. I think that planning ahead, language, and musical abilities also fall out of this same set of neocortical mechanisms, as I've discussed (along with their "free lunch" aspects, thanks to common neural mechanisms) in my earlier books.

SOME READERS MAY HAVE NOTICED BY NOW that this book is not like my previous ones. They were primarily for general readers and only secondarily for fellow scientists, but that order is reversed here. To help compensate, I've provided a glossary starting at page 203 (even the neuroscientists will need it for the brief tutorials in chaos theory and evolutionary biology). Consult it early and often.

And I had the general reader firmly in mind as I did the book design (it's all my fault, even the page layout). The illustrations range from the serious to the sketchy. In *Three Places in New England*, the composer Charles Ives had a characteristic way of playing a popular tune such as "Yankee Doodle" and then dissolving it into his own melody; even a quote of only four notes can be sufficient to release a flood of associations in the listener (something that I tackle mechanistically in *Act II*, when warming up for metaphor mechanisms). As a matter of writer's technique,

I have tried to use captionless thumbnail illustrations as the briefest of scene-setting digressions, to mimic Ives. I have again enlisted the underground architect, Malcolm Wells, to help me out — you won't have any trouble telling which illustrations are Mac's! Furthermore, a painting by the neurobiologist Mark Meyer adorns the cover. For some of my own illustrations, alas, I have had to cope with conveying spatiotemporal patterning in a spatial-only medium (further constrained by being grayscale-only and tree-based!). Although I've relied heavily on musical analogies, the material fairly begs for animations.

I have resisted the temptation to utilize computer simulations, mostly for reasons of clarity (in my own head — and perhaps also the reader's). Simulations, if they are to be more than mere animations of an idea, have hard-to-appreciate critical assumptions. At this stage, simulations are simply not needed — one can comprehend the more obvious consequences of a neocortical Darwin Machine without them, both the modular circuits and the territorial competitions. Plane geometry fortunately suffices, essentially that discovered by the ancient Greeks as they contemplated the hexagonal tile mosaics on the bathhouse floor.

Act I

Everyone knows that in 1859 Darwin demonstrated the occurrence of evolution with such overwhelming documentation that it was soon almost universally accepted. What *not* everyone knows, however, is that on that occasion Darwin introduced a number of other scientific and philosophical concepts that have been of far-reaching importance ever since. These concepts, population thinking and selection, owing to their total originality, had to overcome enormous resistance. One might think that among the many hundreds of philosophers who had developed ideas about change, beginning with the Ionians, Plato and Aristotle, the scholastics, the philosophers of the Enlightenment, Descartes, Locke, Hume, Leibniz, Kant, and the numerous philosophers of the first half of the nineteenth century, that there would have been at least one or two to have seen the enormous heuristic power of that combination of variation and selection. But the answer is no. To a modern, who sees the manifestations of variation and selection wherever he looks, this seems quite unbelievable, but it is a historical fact.

ERNST MAYR, 1994

Looking back into the history of biology, it appears that wherever a phenomenon resembles learning, an instructive theory was first proposed to account for the underlying mechanisms. In every case, this was later replaced by a selective theory. Thus the species were thought to have developed by learning or by adaptation of individuals to the environment, until Darwin showed this to have been a selective process. Resistance of bacteria to antibacterial agents was thought to be acquired by adaptation, until Luria and Delbrück showed the mechanism to be a selective one. Adaptive enzymes were shown by Monod and his school to be inducible enzymes arising through the selection of preexisting genes. Finally, antibody formation that was thought to be based on instruction by the antigen is now found to result from the selection of already existing patterns. It thus remains to be asked if learning by the central nervous system might not also be a selective process, i.e., perhaps learning is not learning either.

NIELS K. JERNE, 1967

1

The Representation Problem and the Copying Solution

Even in the small world of brain science [in the 1860s], two camps were beginning to form. One held that psychological functions such as language or memory could never be traced to a particular region of the brain. If one had to accept, reluctantly, that the brain did produce the mind, it did so as a whole and not as a collection of parts with special functions. The other camp held that, on the contrary, the brain did have specialized parts and those parts generated separate mind functions. The rift between the two camps was not merely indicative of the infancy of brain research; the argument endured for another century and, to a certain extent, is still with us today.

ANTONIO R. DAMASIO, 1995

ONE CELL, ONE MEMORY may not be the way things work, but it seems to be the first way that people think about the problem of locating memories in cells. Even if you aren't familiar with how computers store data, the take-home message of most introductions to the brain is that there are pigeonhole memories — highly specialized interneurons, the firing of which might constitute an item's memory evocation. On the perceptual side of neurophysiology, we call it the *grandmother's face cell* (a neuron that may fire only once a year, at Christmas dinner). On the movement side, if a single interneuron (that's an "insider neuron," neither sensory neuron nor motor neuron) effectively triggers a particular response, it gets called a *command neuron*. In the simplest of arrangements, both would be the same neuron.

Indeed, the Mauthner cells that trigger the escape reflex of the fish are exactly such neurons. If the fish is attacked from one side, the appropriate Mauthner cell fires and a massive tail flip results, carrying the fish away from the nibbles of its predator. Fortunately these cells already had a proper name, so we were spared the *nibble-detector tail-flip cell*.

But we know better than to generalize these special cases to the whole brain — it can't be one cell, one concept. Yet the reasoning that follows isn't as easily recalled as those pigeonhole memory examples that inadvertently become the take-home message from most introductions to the subject. A singular neuron for each concept is rendered implausible in most vertebrates by the neurophysiological evidence that has accumulated since 1928, when the first recordings from sensory nerves revealed a broad range of sensitivity. There were multiple types, with the sensitivity range of one type overlapping that of other types. This overlap, without pure specialties, had been suspected for a long time, at least by the physiologically inclined. Thomas

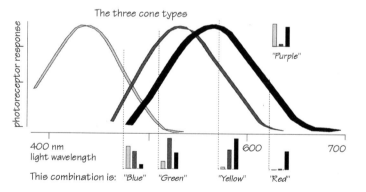

Young formulated his trichromatic theory of colors in 1801; after Hermann von Helmholtz extended the theory in 1865, it was pretty obvious that each special color must be a particular *pattern* of response that was achievable in various ways, not a singular entity. More recently, taste has turned out the same way: bitter is just a pattern of strong and weak responses in four types of taste buds, not the action of a particular type.

This isn't to say that a particular interneuron might not come to specialize in some unique combination — but it's so hard to find narrow specialists, insensitive to all else, that we talk of the expectation of finding one as the "Grandmother's face cell fallacy." The "command neuron" usually comes with scare quotes, too, as the Mauthner cell arrangement isn't a common one. While we seek out the specialized neurons in the hopes of finding a tractable experimental model, we usually recognize that committees are likely the irreducible basis of representations — certainly the more abstract ones we call schemas.

Because the unit of memory is likely to be closely related to sensory and motor schemas, pigeonhole schemes such as one-cell-one-memory had to be questioned. After Karl Lashley got through with his rat cortical lesions and found no crucial neocortical sites for maze memory traces, we had to suspect that a particular "memory trace" was a widespread patterning of some sort, one with considerable redundancy. You're left trying to imagine how a unit of memory could be spatially distributed in a redundant manner, overlapping with other memories.

One technological analogy is the hologram, but the brain seems unlikely to utilize phase information in the same way. A simpler and more familiar example of an ensemble representation is the pattern of lights on a message board. Individually, each light signifies nothing. Only in combination with other lights is there a meaning. More modern examples are the pixels of a computer screen or dot-matrix printer. Back in the 1940s, the physiological psychologist Donald Hebb postulated such an ensemble (which he called a cell-assembly) as the unit of perception — and therefore memory. I'll discuss the interesting history of the cell-assembly in the *Intermission Notes* but for now, just think of one committee–one concept, and that any one cell can serve on multiple committees.

Note that it is not merely the lights which are lit that contain the concept's characteristic pattern: it is just as important that other lights are off, those that might "fog" the desired pattern were they turned on. Fortunately, most neurons of association cortex fire so infrequently that we often take the shortcut of talking only about "activating cells"; in other parts of the nervous system (especially the retina), there are background levels of activity that can be decreased as well as increased (just as gray backgrounds allow the textbook illustrator to use both black and white type) in an analog manner. But, as we shall see, neocortex also has some "digital" aspects.

A minor generalization to Hebb's cell-assembly would be moveable patterns, as when a message board scrolls: the pattern's the thing, irrespective of which cells are used to implement it. I cannot think of any cerebral examples equivalent to the moving patterns of Conway's Game of Life, such as flashers and gliders, but it is well to keep the free-floating patterns of automata in mind.

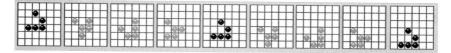

The important augmentation of the message board analogy is a pattern of twinkling lights: the possibility that the relevant memory pattern is a spatiotemporal one, not merely a spatial one. In looking for spatiotemporal patterns and trying to discern components, we are going to have the same problems as the child looking at a large Christmas tree, trying to see the independently flashing strings of lights that have been interwoven.

IN THE LONG RUN, however, a memory pattern cannot be a spatio*temporal* one: long-term memories survive all sorts of temporary shutdowns in the brain's electricity, such as coma; they persist despite all sorts of fogging, such as those occurring with concussions and seizures. Hebb's dual trace memory said that there had to be major representational differences between long-term memory and the more current "working memories," which can be a distinctive pattern of neuron firings. As Hebb put it:

> If some way can be found of supposing that a reverberatory [memory] trace might cooperate with the structural change, and *carry the memory until the growth change is made,* we should be able

to recognize the theoretical value of the trace which is an activity only, without having to ascribe all memory to it.

We are familiar with this archival-versus-current, passive-versus-active distinction from phonograph records, where a spatial-only pattern holds the information in cold storage and a spatiotemporal pattern is recreated on occasion, a pattern almost identical to that which originally produced the spatial pattern. A sheet of music or a roll for a player piano also allows a spatial-only pattern to be converted to a spatiotemporal one. I will typically use musical performance as my spatiotemporal pattern analogy and sheet music as my analogy to a spatial-only underpinning.

At first glimpse, there appear to be some spatial-only sensations, say, those produced by my wristwatch on my skin (it's not really static because I have the usual physiological tremor, and a radial pulse, to interact with its weight). But most of our sensations are more obviously *spatiotemporal*, as when we finger the corner of the page in preparation for turning it. Even if the input appears static, as when we stare at the center of a checkerboard, some jitter is often introduced, as by the small micronystagmus of the eyeball (as I discuss further in the middle of my *Intermission Notes*, the nervous system gets a spatiotemporal pattern from the photoreceptors sweeping back and forth under the image). Whether timeless like a drawing of a comb or changing with time as when feeling a comb running through your hair, the active "working" representation is likely to be spatiotemporal, something like the light sequence in a pinball machine or those winking light strings on the Christmas tree.

Certainly, all of our movements involve spatiotemporal patterns of muscle activation. Even in a static-seeming posture, physiological tremor moves things. In general, the implementation is a spatiotemporal pattern involving many motor neuron pools. Sometimes, as in the case of the fish's tail flip, the command for this starts at one point in time and space, but usually even the *initiation* of the movement schema is spatiotemporal, smeared out in both time and space.

The sensation need not funnel down to a point and then expand outwards to recruit the appropriate response sequence; rather, the spatiotemporal pattern of the sensation could create the appropriate spatiotemporal pattern for the response *without ever having a locus.* Spread out in both time and space, such ephemeral (and perhaps relocatable) ensembles are difficult to summarize in flow charts or metaphors. Think, perhaps, of two voices, one of which (the sensory code) starts the song, is answered by the other voice (movement code); the voices are then intertwined for awhile (and the movement eventually gets underway), and then the second voice finishes the song.

To my mind, the representation problem is *which* spatiotemporal pattern represents a mental object: surely recalling a memory is not a matter of recreating the firing patterns of every cell in the brain, so that they all mimic the activity at the time of input. Some subset must suffice. How big is it? Is it a synchronized ensemble like a chord, as some cortical theories would have it? Or is it more like a single note melody? Or with some chords mixed in? Does it repeat over and over, or does one repetition suffice for a while?

THOSE QUESTIONS WERE IN THE AIR, for the most part, even back in my undergraduate days of the late 1950s, when I first met Hebb after reading his then-decade-old book, *The Organization of Behavior.* Hebb, amazingly, guessed a solution in 1945, even before the first single neuron recordings from mammalian cerebral cortex (glass microelectrodes weren't invented until 1950). Although our data have grown magnificently in recent decades, we haven't improved much on Hebb's statement of the problem, or on his educated guess about where the solution is likely to be found.

> It is inaccurate — worse, it is misleading — to call psychology the study of behavior: It is the study of the underlying processes, just as chemistry is the study of the atom rather than pH values, spectroscopes, and test tubes.
>
> D. O. HEBB, 1980

Multiple microelectrode techniques now allow the sampling of several dozen neurons in a neighborhood spanning a few square millimeters. In motor cortex, even a randomly sampled ensemble can predict which movement, from a standard repertoire, that a trained monkey is about to make. For monkeys forced to wait before acting on a behavioral choice, sustained cell firing during the long hold is mostly up in premotor and prefrontal areas. In premotor and prefrontal cortex, some of the spatiotemporal patterns sampled by multiple microelectrodes are surprisingly precise and task-specific. With the fuzzier imaging techniques, we have recently seen some examples of where work-ing memory patterns might be located: for humans trying to remember telephone numbers long enough to dial them, it's the classical Broca and Wernicke language areas that light up in imaging techniques.

Because recall is so much more difficult than mere recognition (you can recognize an old phone number, even when you can't voluntarily recall it), we may need to distinguish between different representations for the same thing. The cryptographers make a similar distinction between a document and a hashed summary of that document (something like a checksum but capable of detecting even transposed letters). Such a 100-byte "message digest" is capable of recognizing a unique, multipage document ("I've seen that one before") but doesn't contain enough information to actually reconstruct it. So, too, we may have to distinguish between simple Hebbian cell-assemblies — ones that suffice for recognition — and the more detailed ones needed for abstracts and for complete recall.

Hebb's formulation imposes an important constraint on any possible explanation for the cerebral representation: it's got to explain both spatial-only and spatiotemporal patterns, their inter-conversions, their redundancy and spatial extent, their imperfect nature (and characteristic errors therefrom), and the links of assoc-iative memory (including how distortions of old memories are caused by new links). No present technology provides an analogy to help us think about the problem.

THE ROLE OF SIMILAR CONSTRAINTS on theorizing can be seen in how Kepler's three "laws" about planetary orbits posed the gravity problem that Newton went on to solve. Only a half century ago, molecular genetics had a similar all-important constraint that set the stage for a solution. Biologists knew that, whatever the genetic material was, it had to fit inside the cell, be chemically stable — and, most significantly, it had to be capable of making very good copies of itself during cell "division." That posed the problem in a solvable way, as it turned out.

Most people thought that the gene would turn out to be a protein, its three-dimensional nooks and crannies serving as a template for another such giant molecule. The reason Crick and Watson's DNA helical-zipper model caused such excitement in 1953 was because it fit with the copying constraint. It wasn't until a few years later that it became obvious how a triplet of a 4-letter DNA code was translated into strings from the 20-letter amino acid alphabet, and so created enzymes and other proteins.

Looking for molecular copying ability led to the solution of the puzzle of how genes were decoded. Might looking for a neural copying mechanism provide an analogous way of approaching the cerebral code puzzle?

MEMES ARE THOSE THINGS that are copied from mind to mind. Richard Dawkins formulated this concept in 1976 in his book, *The Selfish Gene*. Cell division may copy genes, but minds mimic everything from words to dances. The cultural analog to the gene is the meme (as in mime or mimic); it's the unit of copying. An advertising jingle is a meme. The spread of a rumor is cloning a pattern from one mind to another, the metastasis of a representation.

Might, however, such cloning be seen inside one brain and not just between brains? Might seeing *what* was cloned lead us to the representation, the cerebral code? Copying of an ensemble pattern hasn't been observed yet, but there are reasons to expect it in any brain — at least, in any brain large enough to have a long-distance communications problem.

If the pattern's the thing, how is it transmitted from the left side of the brain to the right side? Or from front to back? We can't send it like a mail parcel, so consider the problems of telecopying, of making a distant copy of a local pattern. Is there a NeuroFax Principle at work?

When tracing techniques were crude, at a millimeter level of resolution, it seemed as if there were point-to-point mappings, an orderly topography for the major sensory pathways such that neighbors remained next to one another. One could imagine that those long corticocortical axon bundles were like fiber optic bundles that convey an image by thousands of little light pipes. But with finer resolution, topographic mappings turn out to be only approximately point-to-point; instead, an axon breaks up into clumps of endings. For the corticocortical axon terminations of the "interoffice mail," this fan-out spans macrocolumnar dimensions and sometimes many millimeters. Exact point-to-point mapping doesn't occur.

Memes are not strung out along linear chromosomes, and it is not clear that they occupy and compete for discrete "loci", or that they have identifiable "alleles" . . . . The copying process is probably much less precise than in the case of genes. . . . Memes may partially blend with each other in a way that genes do not.

RICHARD DAWKINS, 1982

So, at first glimpse, it appears that corticocortical bundles are considerably worse than those incoherent fiber optic bundles that are factory rejects — unless, of course, something else is going on. Perhaps it doesn't matter that the local spatiotemporal pattern is severely distorted at the far end; if codes are arbitrary, why should it matter that there are different codes for *Apple* in different parts of the brain? Just as there are two equally valid roots to a quadratic equation, just as isotopes have identical chemical properties despite different weights, so degenerate codes are quite common. For example, there are six different DNA triplets that all result in leucine being tacked on to a growing peptide.

The main drawback to a degenerate cortical code is that most corticocortical projections are reciprocal: six out of seven interareal pathways have a matching back projection. It might undo the distortion of the forward projection, in the manner of inverse transforms, but that's demanding a lot of careful tuning and regular recalibration. And it isn't simply a matter of each local region having two local codes for *Apple*, one for sending, the other for receiving. Each region has multiple projection targets and thus many possible feedback codes that mean *Apple*.

There might, of course, be some sort of error-correction code that allows a single characteristic spatiotemporal pattern for *Apple*. It would have to remove any distortions caused by the spatial wanderings, plus those associated with temporal dispersions of corticocortical transmission. It would need, furthermore, to operate in both the forward and return paths. I originally dismissed this possibility, assuming that an error-correcting mechanism was too fancy for cerebral circuitry. But, as will become apparent by the end of the following chapter, such error correction is easier than it sounds, thanks to that fanout of the corticocortical axon's terminals contributing to standardization of a spatiotemporal pattern.

COPYING FOR A *FAUX* FAX is going to be needed for cerebral cortex, even if simpler nervous systems, without a long-distance problem, can operate without copying. Copying might also be handy for promoting redundancy. But there is a third reason why copying might have proved useful in a fancy brain: darwinism.

Perhaps it is only a matter of our impoverished knowledge of complex systems, but creativity seems to be a shaping-up process. During the evolution of new species and during the immune response's production of better and better antibodies, successive generations are shaped up, not especially the individual. Yes, the individual is plastic and it learns, but this modification during life is not typically incorporated into the genes that are passed on (learning and experience only change the *chances* of passing on the genes with which one was born — the propensity for learning such things, rather than the things themselves). Yes, culture itself passes along imitations, but memes are easily distorted and easily lost, compared to genuine genes.

Reproduction involves the copying of patterns, sometimes with small chance variations. Creativity may not always be a matter of copying errors and recombination, but it is reasonable to expect that the brain is going to make some use of this elementary darwinian mechanism for editing out the nonsense and emphasizing variations on the better-fitting ones in a next generation.

NATURAL SELECTION ALONE isn't sufficient for evolution, and neither is copying alone — not even copying with selection will suffice. I can identify six essential aspects of the creative darwinian process that bootstraps quality.

1. There must be a reasonably complex pattern involved.
2. The pattern must be copied somehow (indeed, that which is copied may serve to define the pattern).
3. Variant patterns must sometimes be produced by chance.
4. The pattern and its variant must compete with one another for occupation of a limited work space. For example, bluegrass and crab grass compete for back yards.
5. The competition is biased by a multifaceted environment, for example, how often the grass is watered, cut, fertilized, and frozen, giving one pattern more of the lawn than another. That's natural selection.
6. There is a skewed survival to reproductive maturity (environmental selection is mostly juvenile mortality) or a skewed distribution of those adults who successfully mate (sexual selection), so new variants always preferentially occur around the more successful of the current patterns.

With only a few of the six essentials, one gets the more widespread "selective survival" process (which popular usage tends to call darwinian). You may get some changes (evolution, but only in the weakest sense of the word) but things soon settle, running out of steam without the full process to turn the darwinian ratchet.

Indeed, many things called darwinian turn out to have no copying process at all, such as the selective survival of some synaptic connections in the brain during pre- and postnatal development of a single individual. Selective survival, moreover, doesn't even require biology. For example, a shingle beach is one where the waves have carried away the smaller rocks and sand, much as a carving reflects the selective removal of some material to create a pattern. The copying-mutation-selection loop utilized by the small-molecule chemists as they try to demonstrate the power of RNA-based evolution captures most of darwinism, as do "genetic" algorithms of computer science.

Not all of the essentials have to be at the same level of organization. Pattern, copying, and variation involve the genes, but selection is based on the bodies (the phenotypes that carry the genes) and their environment; inheritance, however, is back at the genotype level. In RNA-based evolution, the two levels are combined into one (the RNA serves as a catalyst in a way that affects its survival — but it is also what is copied).

BECAUSE NEURAL VERSIONS OF THE SIX ESSENTIALS are going to play such a large role in the rest of this book, let me comment on the better-known versions for a moment.

The gene is a string of DNA base-pairs that, in turn, instructs the rest of the cell about how to make a protein, perhaps an enzyme that regulates the rate of tissue growth. We'll be looking back from neural implementations, such as movement commands, and trying to see what patterns could have served as the cerebral code to get them going. Larger genetic patterns, such as whole chromosomes, are seldom copied exactly. So, too, we will have to delve below the larger movements to see what the smaller units might be.

While the biological variations seem random, unguided variation isn't really required for a darwinian process to operate. We tend to emphasize randomness for several reasons. First, randomness is the default assumption against which we test claims of guidance. And second, the process will work fine without guidance, without any foreknowledge of a desired result. That said, it might work faster, and in some restricted sense better, with some hints that bias the general direction of the variants; this need not involve anything as fancy as artificial selection. We will see neural versions of random copying errors and recombination, including (in the last chapter) some discussion about how a slow darwinian process might guide a faster one by biasing the general direction in which its variations are done.

Competition between variants depends on some limitation in resources (space in association cortex, in my upcoming examples) or carrying capacity. During a wide-open population explosion, competition is minor because the space hasn't filled up yet.

For competition to be interesting, it must be based on a complex, multifaceted environment. Rather than the environment of grass, we'll be dealing with biases from sensation, feedback from our own movements, and even our moods. Most interestingly, there are both current versions of these environmental factors and memories of past ones.

Many of the offspring have variations that are "worse" than the successful parent pattern but a minority may possess a variant that is an even better fit to the particular multifaceted environment. This tendency to base most new variations on the more successful of the old ones is what Darwin called the principle of inheritance, his great insight and the founding principle of what became population biology.

It means that the darwinian process, as a whole loop, isn't truly random. Rather, it involves repeated exploratory steps where small chance variations are done on well-tested-by-the-environment versions. It's an enormously conservative process, because variations propagate from the base of the most successful adults — not the base of the population as born. Without this proviso, the process doesn't accumulate wisdom about what worked in the past. The neural version also needs exactly the same characteristic, where slight variations are done from an advanced position, not from the original center of the population.

AT LEAST FIVE OTHER FACTORS are known to be important to the evolution of species. The creative darwinian process will run without them, but they affect the stability of its outcome, or the rate of evolution, and will be important for my model of cognitive functions. Just like the catalysts and enzymes that speed chemical reactions without being consumed, they may make improbable outcomes into commonplace ones.

7. Stability may occur, as in getting stuck in a rut (a local peak or basin in the adaptational landscape). Variants occur but they backslide easily. Only particularly large variations can ever escape from a rut, but they are few, and

even more likely to produce nonsense (phenotypes that fail to develop properly, and so die young).

8. Systematic recombination generates many more variants than do copying errors and the far-rarer cosmic-ray mutations. Recombination usually occurs once during meiosis (the grandparent chromosomes are shuffled as haploid sperm and ova are made) and again at fertilization (as the haploid parent genomes are combined into diploid once again, at fertilization). Sex, in the sense of gamete dimorphism (going to the extremes of expensive ova and cheap sperm), was invented several billion years ago and greatly accelerated species evolution over the rate promoted by errors, bacterial conjugation, and retroviruses.

9. Fluctuating environments (seasons, climate changes, diseases) change the name of the game, shaping up more complex patterns capable of doing well in several environments. For such jack-of-all-trades selection to occur, the environment must change much faster than efficiency adaptations can track it, or "lean mean machine" specialists will dominate the expensive generalists.

10. Parcellation, as when rising sea level converts the hilltops of one large island into an archipelago of small islands, typically speeds evolution. This is, in part, because more individuals then live on the margins of the habitat where selection pressure is greater. Also, there is no large central population to buffer change. When rising sea level converted part of the coastline of France into the island of Jersey, the red deer trapped there in the last interglaciation underwent a considerable dwarfing within only a few thousand years.

11. Local extinctions, as when an island population becomes too small to sustain itself, speed evolution because they create empty niches. When subsequent pioneers rediscover the unused resources, their descendants go through a series of generations where there is enough food — even for the more extreme variations that arise, the ones that would ordinarily lose out in the competition with the more optimally endowed, such as the survivors of a resident

population. When the environment again changes, some of those more extreme variants may be able to cope better with the third environment than the narrower range of variants that would reach reproductive age under the regime of a long-occupied niche.

Sexual selection also has the reputation of speeding evolution, and there are "catalysts" acting at several removes, as in Darwin's example of what introducing cats to an English village would do to enhance the bee-dependent flowers, via reducing the rodent populations that disrupt bee hives.

An example of how these catalysts work together is island biogeography, as in the differentiation of Darwin's finches unbuffered by large continental gene pools. Archipelagos allow for many parallel evolutionary experiments. Episodes that recombine the islands (as when sea level falls during an ice age) create winner-take-most tournaments. Most evolutionary change may occur in such isolation, in remote valleys or offshore islands, with major continental populations serving as slowly changing reservoirs that provide pioneers to the chancy periphery.

ALTHOUGH THE CREATIVE DARWINIAN PROCESS will run without these catalysts, using darwinian creativity in a behavioral setting requires some optimization for speed, so that quality is achieved within the time span of thought and action. Accelerating factors are the problem in what the French call *avoir l'esprit de l'escalier* — finally thinking of a witty reply, but only after leaving the party. I will not be surprised if some accelerating factors are almost essential in mental darwinism, simply because of the time windows created by fleeting opportunities.

The wheels of a machine
to play rapidly
must not fit with the utmost exactness
else the attrition diminishes the Impetus.
SIR WALTER SCOTT, discussing Lord Byron's mind

THE NEOCORTICAL PYRAMIDAL NEURON

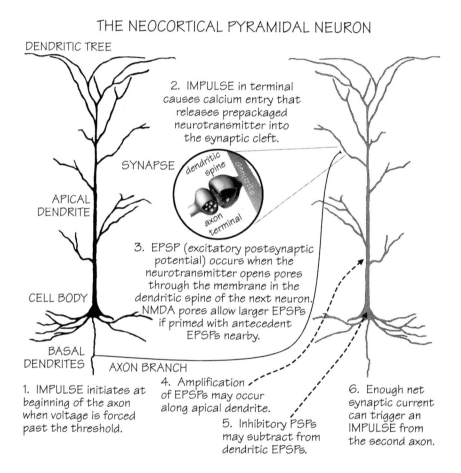

DENDRITIC TREE

2. IMPULSE in terminal causes calcium entry that releases prepackaged neurotransmitter into the synaptic cleft.

SYNAPSE

dendritic spine

dendrite

axon terminal

APICAL DENDRITE

3. EPSP (excitatory postsynaptic potential) occurs when the neurotransmitter opens pores through the membrane in the dendritic spine of the next neuron. NMDA pores allow larger EPSPs if primed with antecedent EPSPs nearby.

CELL BODY

BASAL DENDRITES

AXON BRANCH

1. IMPULSE initiates at beginning of the axon when voltage is forced past the threshold.

4. Amplification of EPSPs may occur along apical dendrite.

5. Inhibitory PSPs may subtract from dendritic EPSPs.

6. Enough net synaptic current can trigger an IMPULSE from the second axon.

2

Cloning in Cerebral Cortex

All scribes, however careful, are bound to make a few errors,
and some are not above a little willful "improvement." If they
all copied from a single master original, meaning would not be
greatly perverted. But let copies be made from other copies,
which in their turn were made from other copies, and errors
will start to become cumulative and serious. We tend to regard
erratic copying as a bad thing, and in the case of human
documents it is hard to think of examples where errors can be
described as improvements. I suppose the scholars of the
Septuagint could at least be said to have started something big
when they mistranslated the Hebrew word for "young woman"
into the Greek word for "virgin," coming up with the prophecy:
"Behold a virgin shall conceive and bear a son. . . ." Anyway,
as we shall see, erratic copying in biological replicators can in a
real sense give rise to improvement, and it was essential for the
progressive evolution of life that some errors were made.
RICHARD DAWKINS, *The Selfish Gene*, 1976

THIS IS THE HARDEST CHAPTER in the whole book. In it, I have
to delve into the neuroanatomy and neurophysiology of
cortical neurons, importing lessons from such seemingly
unrelated subjects as synchronously flashing fireflies. By the end
of this chapter, I will have shown how copying could arise in
neocortex. By the end of the sixth chapter, the cortical equivalents
of all the darwinian essentials and all the accelerating factors will

have been examined. But it gets easier, not harder, starting with the fourth chapter.

Neurophysiologists distinguish between cell properties and circuit properties, much as biologists distinguish between genotype and phenotype. Some phenomena are clearly due to the circuit rather than the cells involved, to the wiring rather than the components — a new property "emerges" from the particular combination. You won't find it in any one neuron. The classical example of an emergent property involves lateral inhibition and it is the reason that Keffer Hartline got a Nobel Prize in 1967.

Thanks to local activity contributing to a ring of depression in surrounding neurons, lateral inhibition sharpens up fuzzy boundaries. Compound eyes, the many narrow-angle photoreceptors of which provide an extreme case of fuzzy optics, have a series of inhibitory interconnections that are capable of recreating a light-dark boundary in the environment, restoring much of what was lost.

But lateral inhibition also has a tendency to produce features where none exist, illusions such as the Mach bands that you see if looking through a narrow slit between your fingers. Georg von Békésy, whose studies of such sideways interactions in the cochlea were the subject of his 1961 Nobel Prize, also produced illusions from skin surfaces, to illustrate the generality of the lateral inhibition principles. Antagonistic surrounds ("Mexican hats") 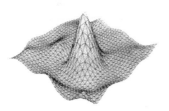 are common in all the first half-dozen stages of the analysis of a visual image, though they become somewhat elongated and asymmetric ("Australian bush hats") in primary visual cortex. Because of the many axon collaterals that branch laterally in neocortex, lateral inhibition extends several millimeters.

Both the sharpening of fuzzy boundaries and the illusions are emergent properties of a laterally inhibiting neural network. What might be the emergent consequences of lateral *excitation*?

THERE IS GOOD REASON to worry about recurrent excitation. It is potentially regenerative, in the same sense as a string of fire

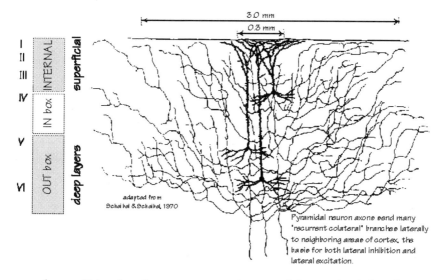

Pyramidal neuron axons send many "recurrent collateral" branches laterally to neighboring areas of cortex, the basis for both lateral inhibition and lateral excitation.

crackers. It is also the most prominent wiring principle of mammalian neocortex.

A few words about cerebral cortex, the icing on the brain's cake: in this cake, it's the frosting that has the appearance of layering! Six layers are usually identified on the basis of cell size

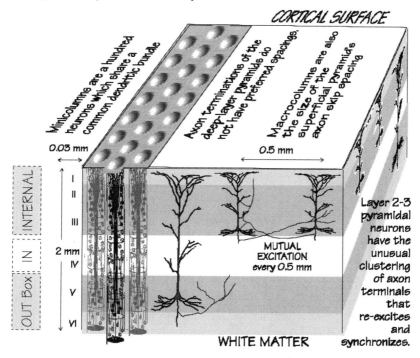

or axon packing density, though we sometimes subdivide it further (in primary visual cortex, one talks about layers 4a, 4b, 4cα, and 4cβ). At other times, we lump layers together: when I mention the "superficial layers," I'm combining layers 1, 2, and 3.

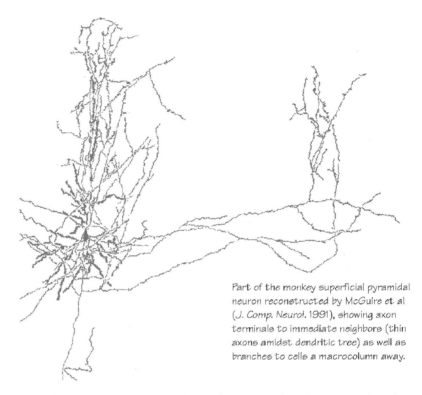

Part of the monkey superficial pyramidal neuron reconstructed by McGuire et al (*J. Comp. Neurol.* 1991), showing axon terminals to immediate neighbors (thin axons amidst dendritic tree) as well as branches to cells a macrocolumn away.

Furthermore, there are three functional groupings that have become apparent: on the analogy to the mail boxes stacked on many a desk, layer 4 could be said to be the *IN* box of neocortex, because most of the inputs from the thalamus terminate there. The deep layers could be called the *OUT* box, as pyramidal neurons of layers 5 and 6 send axons outside the cortex, back to thalamus or down to the spinal cord, and so forth. The neurons of the superficial layers seem to constitute the *INTERNAL* mailbox of the neocortex, specializing in the interoffice memos. Interactions among the superficial pyramidal neurons are what this book is mostly about, as these neurons seem capable of implementing a darwinian copying competition, one that can shape up quality from humble beginnings.

The axons of the superficial pyramidal cells are prominent in the corpus callosum and other long corticocortical paths, but also in the intrinsic horizontal connections: those axon branches that never leave the superficial layers because they run sideways. They preferentially terminate on other superficial pyramidal neurons — and in a patterned manner, too. Some axon branches go to near neighbors, but the ones that go further ignore a whole series of intermediate neurons before communicating with those about 0.5 mm distant.

Those sparsely populated gaps are something like the Sherlock Holmes story about the dog that didn't bark in the night. It took a long time before anyone noticed this fact. In 1975 came the first hint of these gap patterns. In 1982, when Jennifer Lund and Kathleen Rockland first studied the gaps in the superficial layers' intrinsic horizontal connections, it was in the visual cortex of the tree shrew. Though the gap distance varies, we now know that it is a common arrangement for many areas of neocortex, and for many animal species. Thanks to the detailed reconstructions of several HRP-injected superficial pyramidal neurons by Barbara McGuire and her colleagues, we also know that these synaptic connections are likely to be excitatory, probably using glutamate as their neurotransmitter, and that their predominant targets are other superficial pyramidal neurons.

Their axons have dozens of branches, going sideways in many radial directions, fanning out eventually into thousands of axon terminals. Although no single superficial pyramidal neuron has enough terminals to fill in a doughnut, we might expect a small minicolumn group of such neurons to produce a ring of excitation, as well as the central spot of excitation from the branches to immediate neighbors. Point-to-area is the more common arrangement for axon projections, such as those of the pyramidal neurons of the deep layers. Recurrent inhibition is also seen, but only the recurrent excitation of the superficial layers of neocortex has this Sherlock-Holmes feature of prominent silent gaps.

Optical imaging techniques that look down on the brain's surface are now capable of resolving a spread of activity in cortex. Stimulation of a restricted area of retina, of a type that classically would be expected to concentrate cortical activity in only one area

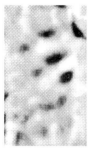 of the exposed cortical surface, is now seen to contribute to multiple hot spots of activity at macrocolumnar separations, much as predicted.

The neocortical versions of long-term potentiation (LTP) are also concentrated in the superficial layers. We know that *N*-methyl-D-aspartate (NMDA) types of postsynaptic receptors, which have the unusual characteristic of augmenting their strength when inputs arrive in clusters (such as quasi-synchronously from different sources), are especially common in the superficial layers.

All of this raises the possibility of self-reexciting loops, not unlike the reverberating circuits postulated for the spinal cord by Rafael Lorente de Nó in 1938, in the very first volume of the *Journal of Neurophysiology*. If the synaptic strengths are high enough, and the paths long enough to escape the refractory periods that would otherwise limit re-excitation, closed loops of activity ought to be possible, impulses chasing their tails. Moshe Abeles, whose Jerusalem lab often observes more than a dozen cortical neurons at a time, has seen some precise impulse timing of one neuron, relative to another, in premotor and prefrontal cortex neuron ensembles. It is unknown whether or not these firing patterns represent reverberation, in Lorente's original sense of recirculating loops. These long, precisely-timed firing patterns are important for the notion of spatiotemporal patterns that I will later develop.

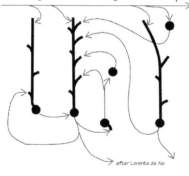

branching axon activating cortical loops

after Lorente de No

EMERGENT SYNCHRONY is well known as a commonplace consequence of recurrent excitation, one that ought to be seen with even weak connection strengths and short paths In 1665, the Dutch physicist Christiaan Huygens noticed that two pendulum clocks hanging from a common support were synchronized. When he disturbed the synchrony, it returned within a half hour. Harmonic oscillators are slower to entrain than nonlinear relaxation oscillators, which can take just a few cycles.

The most famous example of entrainment is probably menstrual cycles in women's dormitories. More dramatic in appearance is a whole tree filled with little lights, flashing in unison. No, I don't mean a Christmas tree wired up, under the control of a single flasher — there's a natural, wireless example based on hundreds of independent oscillators. The little lights are hundreds of fireflies, and they have no leader to set the pace.

> Imagine a tree thirty-five to forty feet high, apparently with a firefly on every leaf, and all the fireflies flashing in perfect unison at a rate of about three times in two seconds, the tree being in complete darkness between flashes. Imagine a tenth of a mile of river front with an unbroken line of mangrove trees with fireflies on every leaf flashing in synchronization, the insects on the trees at the ends of the line acting in perfect unison with those between. Then, if one's imagination is sufficiently vivid, he may form some conception of this amazing spectacle.

It doesn't require any elaborate notions of mimicry to account for the firefly entrainment; even small tendencies to advance to the next flash when stimulated with light will suffice to create a "rush hour." Furthermore, you usually do not see waves propagating through such a population, except perhaps when the flashing is just beginning or ending. Even in cortical simulations with propagation delays, near-synchrony is seen, in much the way (anomalous dispersion) that some velocities can exceed the speed of light.

Weak mutual re-excitation (a few percent of threshold) is quite sufficient to entrain; one need not postulate strong connection strengths in the manner needed for Lorente's recirculating chains. So long as the neurons (or fireflies) already have enough input to fire repeatedly, there will be an entrainment tendency if they mutually re-excite one another. And that is exactly what superficial pyramidal neurons, 0.5 mm apart, seem so likely to do. The triple combination — mutual re-excitation, silent gaps that focus it, and the resulting entrainment tendencies — is what gives the superficial layers of neocortex the potential of being a Darwin Machine.

LOOKING DOWN FROM ON HIGH at the superficial layers of neocortex, in what the neuroanatomists call "tangential slices," is like looking down on a forest from a balloon. Any one neuron is seen in a top-down perspective, orthogonal to that seen from the side in the usual surface-to-depth slice. Like the branches of any one tree, any one neuron has a dendritic tree, but also an axon tree, much as the forest's tree has branching roots below ground.

The axon of a single superficial pyramidal neuron will be seen to spread in many directions. Though sensory neurons and motor neurons may vary, the average interneuron sends out as many synapses as it receives, usually between 2,000 and 10,000. Not enough radial plots have yet been done to know how symmetric the horizontal spread is, but it seems clear that the axon branches travel in many directions from the cell.

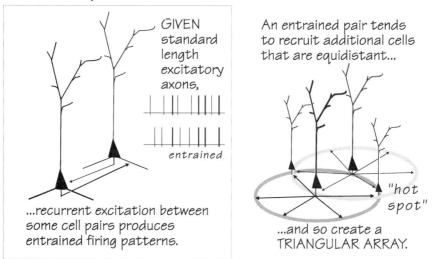

GIVEN standard length excitatory axons,

entrained

...recurrent excitation between some cell pairs produces entrained firing patterns.

An entrained pair tends to recruit additional cells that are equidistant...

"hot spot"

...and so create a TRIANGULAR ARRAY.

The distance from the cell body to the center of the axon terminal cluster, studied mostly in the side views, is not the same in all cortical areas. That "0.5 mm" mentioned earlier is really as small as 0.4 mm (in primary visual cortex of monkeys) or as large as 0.85 mm (in sensorimotor cortex). It scales with the width of the basal dendritic tree. I'll use 0.5 mm as my standard example of this local metric; it corresponds to a basal dendritic tree of about 0.25

mm spread, which is also about the spread of one cluster of axon terminals and the extent of one silent gap.

If two superficial pyramidal neurons, about 0.5 mm apart, are interested in the same features because of similar inputs and thresholds, their spike trains ought to start exhibiting occasional spike synchrony. It need not be all the spikes from each neuron for the following analysis to be relevant; only some of their spikes need synchronize via the recurrent excitation.

There should also be some minor tendency for two such cells, already firing repeatedly, to recruit another cell 0.5 mm away that is almost active. If that third superficial pyramidal neuron becomes active, we should see three often-synchronized neurons forming an equilateral triangle. But that is not the end of it: there is a second site receiving synchronous input from the parent pair (this is exactly like that elementary exercise in plane geometry where a compass is used to bisect a line or drop a perpendicular). So a fourth neuron might join the chorus.

And because the third and fourth cells provide new annuli of excitation, either can combine with one of the first pair to bring a fifth point into synchrony. What we have, it is apparent, is a mechanism for forming up a triangular array of some size, nodes of synchronized activity 0.5 mm from corresponding cells of this chorus. It could work either by synchronizing preexisting activity or by recruiting otherwise sub-threshold neurons at the nodes. Once a potential node is surrounded by a few synchronous nodes exciting it, there ought to be a hot spot, an unusually effective con-vergence of simultaneous inputs.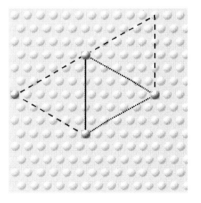

This triangular array annexa-tion tendency is not unlimited. (Regions with insufficiently excited neurons, as I discuss in the latter part of chapter 6, provide *barriers* to any further empire-building.) And the triangular array is surely ephemeral, here now and gone in seconds. When it is shut

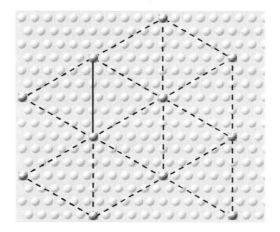

down by enough inhibition (or reduction of excitation), it will be as if a blackboard had been erased.

Traces will linger, however, in much the way that blackboards retain ghostly images of former patterns. The synaptic strengths should remain changed for a while; indeed, the synchrony-sensitive long-term potentiation of the superficial neocortical layers suggests that synaptic strength can remain augmented for many minutes. This will make it easier to recreate the active form of the triangular array — perhaps not all of its spatial extent, but part of it.

THE LATTICE CONNECTIVITY seen in the anatomy, it should be said, does not fall into neat triangular arrays, measured by distance in the tangential plane of section. Though the neuroanatomists speak of "polka-dot" patterns and "lattices" for the axon terminal clusters in the superficial layers, the spacing of the clusters is only roughly triangular. Of course, adjusting conduction velocity or synaptic delay during a tune-up period could make a triangular array, when replotted as "driving time" rather than distance.

But not even an equal conduction time, for converging simultaneously on a potential recruit, is actually required for the present theory. Though exact synchrony has been convenient for introducing the principles, all that triangular arrays require in the long run is a prenatal tune-up period that results in a good-enough self-organization, so that most of the six surrounding nodes produce axon clusters that mutually overlap in a manner that aids entrainment. It may not matter to this self-organizing principle what an external observer would find "regular." I'll stick to triangular array terminology for the theory, but don't expect to find exact triangles in either the anatomy or physiology, only good-enough approximations.

FROM A PAIR OF LIKE-MINDED CELLS, we see the possibility of a large chorus, all singing in synchrony. Furthermore, it's a chorus that can recruit additional members out on its edges. Like a choir standing on risers, these singers tend to space themselves so that each is standing in between two singers on the row below. The choir isn't as perfect a triangular array as the fruit displays at your corner grocery, but it's a good enough approximation to the familiar packing principle.

So far, this choir only chants in unison. It's monomaniacal, perhaps only interested in one feature of the stimulus. It's surely not the true Hebbian cell-assembly. The choir corresponding to a concept representation would surely sing in parts, just as sopranos carry one melody and the altos another, each group having different interests. We will need polyphony for harmonious categories, not just chants.

The purpose of art is to lay bare the questions
which have been hidden by the answers.

JAMES BALDWIN

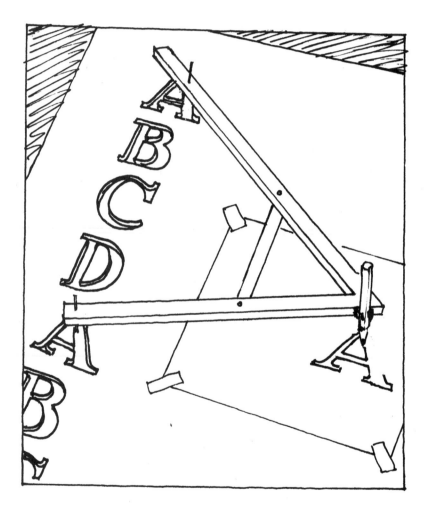

3

A Compressed Code Emerges

These self-re-exciting systems [cell-assemblies] could
not consist of one circuit of two or three neurons, but
must have a number of circuits. . . . I could assume
that when a number of neurons in the cortex are
excited by a given sensory input they tend to become
interconnected, some of them at least forming a
multicircuit closed system. . . . The idea then [1945]
was that a *percept* consists of assemblies excited
sensorily, a *concept* of assemblies excited centrally, by
other assemblies.

D. O. HEBB, 1980

POLYPHONIC MUSIC elaborated on chants by combining a
number of independent but harmonizing melodies. The
task of this chapter is considerably easier: we only have to
combine notes, each from a different triangular array, into a
simple melody (polyphony, as chapter 7 will show, is a useful
analogy to what's going on in category representations). While
this chapter starts with some issues regarding the cortical
landscape from which the choir sings, it soon progresses to an
abstraction much like written music.

Happily, by the end of this chapter, we will see the choir
coalesce into sections, each of which sings the complete song.
Unlike the placements favored by choirmasters, the sopranos are
not grouped together; it's more like each section has one soprano,
one alto, one bass, and so forth, each singing a different part. Each

section is surrounded by neighbors, sections that are similarly diverse. You might think that this would make it difficult for a choirmaster — if one exists — to conduct, but remember that string quartets get along nicely without a conductor, and what I will describe here is a chorus of string quartets.

In cortex, it looks as if one string-quartet section occupies a space that is hexagonal in shape and about 0.5 mm across. It could constitute the most elementary version of Hebb's cell-assembly, one that could represent a word, a face, or a pronunciation. Cloning indeed clues us in, suggesting what the relevant code might be — that characteristic pattern needed for the first darwinian essential. To get there, however, we first need to consider a few more aspects of the geometry and its relevant neurophysiology.

THE "HOT SPOT" COULD BE SIZEABLE, because of the width of those 0.25 mm clusters of terminals. But the history of neurophysiology suggests that, functionally speaking, the hot spot might be far smaller, perhaps as small as a minicolumn (0.03 mm diameter, and a small percent of the area). Before returning to the spatial extent of a triangular array, let us consider the size of its nodes (I'll use node as a punctate theoretical term, with hot spot referring to physiologists measure, and axon terminal clusters referring to what anatomists see).

Anatomical connectivity (the fanout of the axon terminals, the width of dendritic trees) is usually far more widespread than physiological responsiveness (such as receptive field centers). Indeed, at a few removes, every neuron in the brain can potentially connect to every other neuron — but such extensive funneling rarely happens. Antagonistic surrounds serve to concentrate things. In the retina, for example, wide areas of the photoreceptor mosaic would seem to have paths to a second-order cell, but a bipolar cell usually has a far smaller receptive field center, thanks to flanking inhibition (or it has an inhibited center with flanking excitation, the other type of antagonistic center-surround arrangement commonly seen) except during dark adaptation.

In addition to antagonistic arrangements, some axon terminals seem to have very weak synaptic strengths; indeed, we sometimes talk of "silent synapses." Anatomically, they're there; physiologically, they're undetectable most of the time. An example of this second type of physiological focusing is the projection from a thalamic neuron, one specializing in just one finger tip, to the hand map in cerebral cortex. Its axon terminal branches seem to span much of the hand's map, but, when you look at the cortical neurons they're feeding, you find that they typically have small receptive fields, little larger than those of thalamic neurons. Another indicator of size: visual cortex cells at millimeter separations with similar orientation preference are interconnected, suggesting the possibility of hot spots that are as small as those 0.03 mm minicolumns.

The superficial pyramidal neurons are not the only cells contacted by the intrinsic axon collaterals; about 20 percent of the axon terminals are onto smooth stellate neurons (that themselves produce GABAergic inhibition), presumably contributing to forms of flanking inhibition that reduce the size of the hot spot.

THERE SHOULD BE A MARKED STABILITY of the triangular arrays formed by the hot spots, even under various perturbations. Let us suppose that a triangular array is firing in a repeated cycle. And that one point in the midst of a triangular array tries to fire out of sync, later than its neighbors.

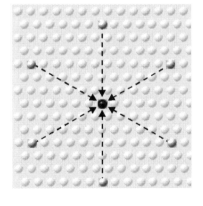

It has, however, six neighbors that are all sending it synchronous inputs at the standard time in the cycle, thus tending to correct it (actually, it may have a dozen because the axons tend to have several terminal clusters 0.5 mm apart). The same argument applies if the idiosyncratic neuron attempts to omit a impulse. Similarly, early firings tend to be corrected the next time around if the neuron has any tendency to produce longer-than-average interimpulse intervals following an earlier-than-average impulse.

Spatially, there is the aforementioned tendency to focus synchronous excitation on the center of the hot spot. What both tendencies mean is that, like a crystal forming, we might expect to see some standardization. One might almost think of it as error correction.

Another force for standardization may be the minicolumn of association cortex (represented as a raised bump in many of my "tangential slice" illustrations), those hundred cells organized around a dendritic bundle. The well-studied orientation columns of primary visual cortex seem to prefer similar stimuli, and the superficial pyramidal neurons have many close-in axon collaterals before the silent gap that often excite near neighbors. These suggest that a number of the minicolumn's 39 superficial pyramidal neurons may be synchronously activated. Because of this, I have not found it useful to distinguish between the individual superficial pyramidal neuron and all the superficial pyramidal neurons within a given minicolumn. The six neighbors could be as many as 39x6=234 superficial pyramidal neurons, speaking together to exact conformity.

One may thus think of the "cells" and "nodes" as really work-alike minicolumns. This tendency to act as a group could eliminate the "holes" in the lattice that might otherwise result from the incomplete "polka-dot" annuli of an individual superficial pyramidal neuron, and give rise to the point-to-annulus property that I infer.

DOES A HOT SPOT FORM at precisely the location suggested by the node of a triangular array? It need not, of course, if other wiring principles override the triangular tendency; for example, making connections with other orientation columns of the same orientation angle might obscure triangular tendencies in primary visual cortex. But this is a theory for association cortex, not for the most specialized of cortical areas. Clustered recurrent excitatory terminals have indeed been found in many neocortical areas of many animal species.

Any one superficial pyramidal neuron's annulus isn't perfect, of course, because its terminal clusters do not provide full coverage. But when six minicolumn's worth of them overlap at the same node (even more, actually, because of the tendency of the axon to continue across another silent gap to produce another cluster), there will be one point that will have more input than others, and this ought to help define the node more narrowly. Furthermore, the cells implementing surround inhibition in the superficial layers of neocortex, the large stellate cells, have axons that reach far enough (except in rats) — so six inhibitory point-to-area circles also help define a node via subtraction.

As we shall see in the next chapter, some synaptic augmentation mechanisms, such as those at the NMDA synapses, are available for rewarding such convergence. The NMDA synapses have a remarkably imprecise notion of synchrony, so augmentation per se might not be sensitive to the equal conduction distances that define the triangle. Exact synchrony of synaptic potentials depends on identical conduction times, all else being equal. Yet ordinary spatial summation — one bump standing on the shoulder of another postsynaptic potential — can define synchrony with considerable precision if the threshold for impulse production can be exceeded only by the optimal overlap, peak atop peak. Higher thresholds will shrink the size of hot spots and, if the conduction speeds are equal, center them equidistant from their inputs.

LET US NOW CONSIDER THE ENSEMBLE PROBLEM in the context of this tendency to recruit a triangular chorus. We don't have just one triangular array, but multiple ones that interdigitate.

When looking at a banana, various types of feature detectors ought to be interested; let us say that the parents of one triangular array (**A**) are fans of the yellow color of the banana. Other superficial pyramidal neurons will likely be interested in one or another of the tangents to the banana's profile, and so one might get another triangular array (**B**) forming up to specialize in horizonal line representation. This second *horizontal* array need not be synchronized with the *yellow* array (as a common form of the binding theory assumes) for present purposes.

Furthermore, the horizontal-tangent's array might start several millimeters away from where the yellow array starts. One can easily imagine a half-dozen separate features, each with its own triangular array, each starting from a different part of the cortical work space. Provided that each array starts up on the same slant (this assumption will become more reasonable once we discuss evoking memories via resonances), the various triangular arrays will be parallel to one another.

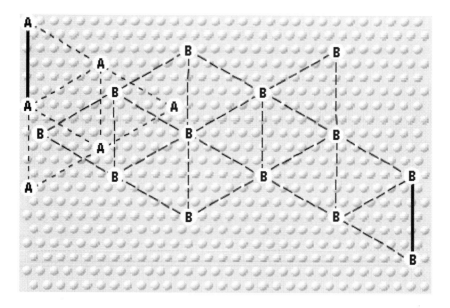

IS THE HEBBIAN CELL-ASSEMBLY the whole collection of triangular arrays, each stretching over many millimeters, looking like those multiple strings of Christmas tree lights, out of sync with one another but flashing together within strings?

No, because that ensemble isn't the minimal cell-assembly that could contain the minimal information needed to reconstruct it. There is obviously lots of redundancy in such a repetitive set of triangular arrays. Let us imagine using an unusually capable microscope and increasing the magnification as we gaze down on the cortical surface. Fewer and fewer nodes of each triangular array will be included as we increase the mag, just as zooming in on a flashing Christmas tree will encompass fewer and fewer lights in sync.

Eventually we will zoom a bit too far, so that one of the triangular arrays (say, *yellow*) will no longer have a representative in our field of view. We might notice this because there are no longer any synchronous spots. So we zoom back out a little and one member of the *yellow* chorus pops back into sight. It's now about 0.5 mm across our field of view. We decrease the mag a little further and now we're seeing several sets of synchronized spots.

So is the minimal Hebbian cell-assembly contained within a 0.5 mm circle? No, it is actually a hexagon, one that is 0.5 mm between parallel sides. We can suppose that we have, lining an edge of such a hexagon, one representative from each of *N* triangular arrays. Move the *N*th array (say, the *yellow* specialists) out a little and other *yellow* point will creep into the opposite side of our original hexagon. It's just like screen wrap on your computer monitor, where a line "ends around." While the Hebbian cell-assembly may not look like a hexagon, its spatial extent may not be any larger than a hexagon, thanks to The Wrap.

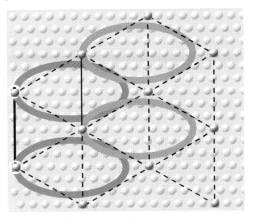

The cells activated by an object were intentionally made to lay on an ellipse of about 0.8 mm width

in cortex, so as to be larger than the 0.5 mm axon gap. But since each point on the ellipse creates its own triangular array (only one is shown), they "end-around" and demonstrate that a 0.5 mm hexagon is the "unit area" of non-redundant points.

WHAT'S THE RELATIONSHIP between hexagonal mosaics and the triangular arrays? There are some potential confusions, particularly because of the similarity in dimensions, each being about 0.5 mm (as are macrocolumns, which are areas with similar sources of distant inputs). The hexagon is a committee comprised of one member from each of a number of different triangular arrays.

Because a hexagon is the largest nonredundant collection of points from a set of triangular arrays, the hexagon is a shorthand term that we must treat with care, lest we become overly concrete.

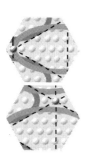

For example, that the largest nonrepeating area is a hexagon does not tell us that it is a *fixed* hexagon. Our hexagonal-shaped viewing mask can be moved about (though not rotated) and still fulfill the requirement of containing only one element of each triangular array. If you try this exercise with your wallpaper, remember that checkerboards are the other common regular mosaic; we're unlikely to encounter square mosaics here because there is no apparent copying mechanism for them.

We might still see hexagons embedded in the anatomy if something in the underlying cortical circuitry tended to make some areas interact as groups. The immovable color blobs might serve as fixed anchors, as might the macrocolumns (ocular dominance columns also span about 0.5 mm). Perhaps the **ABCD** points tend to form an emergent rhythm that comes to be contained in the local connectivity. It, then, would have a territorial identity that would make some mask placements more meaningful than others — an *anchored* hexagon.

The Wrap has an interesting consequence for the issue of what's the unit pattern (still a problem in biology; see Helena Cronin's answer in the glossary under "gene"): even if the feature detectors that were originally active were scattered over a few

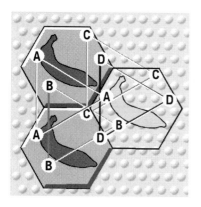

millimeters, we now have a more compact representation. *We have compacted the presynchronization, premosaic Hebbian cell-assembly into a small standard space,* presumably making it easier to restart the characteristic spatiotemporal firing pattern from a local cortical circuit; indeed, any of a number of similar hexagons could proceed to clone a whole population of the resurrected spatiotemporal pattern.

Of course, we have a tendency to concentrate on only those cells that are firing in response to the banana. If you also consider what cells must remain silent to avoid fogging the characteristic pattern, the cerebral code for *Banana* occupies the full hexagon. In the musical analogy that opened this chapter, this hexagon corresponds to the string quartet. Its members, too, have to know when to keep quiet so as not to ruin the harmony.

Another way to look at the unit-pattern problem is to ask what is the minimum cell-assembly needed to reignite this spatio-temporal pattern. That's the minimal assembly of cells which can begin to generate a hexagonal mosaic, not necessarily all the individual "tiles" of the parent pattern stretching out laterally across a cortical work space, but at least a "starter" fraction of it. Because it takes two cells 0.5 mm apart to start generating a triangular array, the minimal Hebbian cell-assembly is two adjacent hexagons worth of the characteristic spatiotemporal pattern. Even if sensory input isn't providing a subliminal fringe of almost-active inputs for triangular node recruitment to boost, the NMDA augmentation can still recruit a new node; it just takes longer than if sensory input was already pushing the nodal neurons into the subthreshold region. In chapter 5, I will

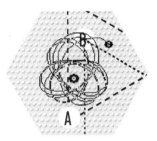

Two triangular arrays may, if maintained long enough, alter synaptic strengths, creating attractors (here simulated with two magnets attracting a pendulum) within a hexagon's circuitry that will sustain the firing pattern.

elaborate on the reconstitution of spatiotemporal firing patterns from spatial-only connectivity patterns and revisit this point.

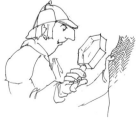

For now, observe that our original collection of feature detectors, possibly scattered over some distance in cortex, has become rather like those hexagonal mosaics forming the floors of the Grecian steam

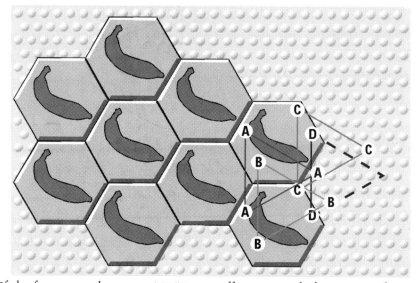

If the four triangular arrays ABCD are sufficient to code for *Banana*, then we have a clone of *Banana* when another complete set of ABCD points is successfully recruited. Hexagonal mosaics are secondary to sets of triangular arrays.

baths 2,500 years ago. Looking down on the cortex with fine enough resolution won't necessarily reveal the boundaries of even anchored hexagons — not any more than you can detect the boundaries of the unit pattern of wallpaper in the midst of the mosaic it forms. But looking down on the cortical surface ought to reveal a triangular array via its synchrony, and then another such triangular array offset somewhat in time. Perhaps we would see one triangular array, and then the others, recruit additional territory. It would be as if additional hexagonal tiles were being added to the unfinished floor. Later we might see the finished portion of the tiling retreat, fading out as if erased, or perhaps replaced by a competing string-quartet pattern, advancing from the other direction.

The recurrent excitation of the superficial layers of neocortex seems an excellent setup for cloning spatiotemporal patterns. Like the patches of bluegrass and crabgrass in my backyard, they could even compete for territory, though at the expense of losing their clonelike uniformity near the cerebral frontiers.

The purpose of art is to lay bare the questions
which have been hidden by the answers.

JAMES BALDWIN

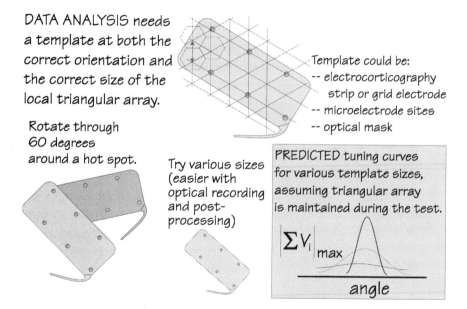

DATA ANALYSIS needs
a template at both the
correct orientation and
the correct size of the
local triangular array.

Template could be:
-- electrocorticography
   strip or grid electrode
-- microelectrode sites
-- optical mask

Rotate through
60 degrees
around a hot spot.

Try various sizes
(easier with
optical recording
and post-
processing)

PREDICTED tuning curves
for various template sizes,
assuming triangular array
is maintained during the test.

$$\left.\sum V_i\right|_{max}$$

angle

SOME EXPERIMENTAL STRATEGIES
FOR DETECTING TRIANGULAR ARRAYS

4

Managing the Cerebral Commons

[Jorge Luis Borges] talked of a country that prided
itself on its cartographical institute and the excellence
of its maps. As the years went by, this institute would
draw maps of greater and greater accuracy until at last
the institute achieved the ultimate, the full-scale map.
And, Borges says, if you wander through the desert
today, you can see places where portions of the map are
still pegged to the region they represent!

MICHAEL A. ARBIB, 1985

THE MAP IS NOT THE TERRITORY, as various people said earlier
in the century, but Arbib goes on to emphasize that our job
as brain theorists is *not* to replace a "life richly lived by the
running of some computer program." We've got to extract something simpler, a maplike guide to the underlying complexity,
despite the seeming functional incomprehensibility of those cells
in the hidden layers in connectionist networks. We need brain
abstractions — such as common processes, used again and again
— in order to appreciate the fine details.

Among the abstractions that have recently been helpful are
those six essentials of a darwinian process: a *characteristic pattern*
that is *copied*, occasional *variants* that *compete* for a work space,
with success biased by a multifaceted *environment*, and with the
more successful producing most of the next round of slight
variants (Darwin's *inheritance principle*). In the last chapter, we
saw how copying mechanisms also helped identify a characteristic

pattern. The predicted mosaics of electrical activity are just one ephemeral state of the cerebral cortex, but they may provide a guide to what else it does. If we can learn to think about the dynamically reforming patchwork quilt of cloning territories as simply as we think about maps, perhaps we can find a way around the hidden-layer incomprehensibility.

This chapter (far easier than the last two) will address the variant patterns and the work space itself, and later chapters will consider cloning competitions in more detail. In between is some chaos, in the best sense of the word, that underlies the memorized environment. But first we are going to need some metaphors to guide us in exploring a jack-of-all-trades work space. We need a lot of multifunctional potential (potentially powerful, but it makes it difficult to name things) rather than a lot of fixed compartments.

WE HUMANS HAVE A LOT OF CEREBRAL CORTEX, enough to cover four sheets of typing paper; that's the potential size of our patchwork quilt of competing hexagonal patterns. A chimpanzee's cerebral cortex is equally thick but there's only enough, when all is flattened out, to cover one sheet of paper. 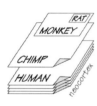 Monkeys have about a postcard worth, and rats are down in postage stamp territory. So far, after a century of neuroscience, there's nothing to suggest that a square millimeter worth of human cortex is much different than the same area in a monkey's brain.

But, though everyone assumes that bigger is likely better, we've had trouble saying in what way that four times as much cortex has been better. There are increases everywhere in the forebrain structures during the evolution from apes to humans. Yes, there are some human abilities such as language, music, planning ahead, accurate throwing, and toolmaking that might require some additional cortical space beyond that available in the apes, but they haven't been "tacked on" as a bulge here and a bump there, in the way a house is often enlarged over the years.

It seems to be easier to increase all of cortex than just to selectively enlarge one piece. This wouldn't have surprised Charles Darwin, who emphasized specialized adaptations but also acknowledged that the underlying variations often involved quite general aspects of growth and form, inextricably linking some functions. Many of the new or improved-beyond-the-apes human skills seem to share cortical space with one another, allowing for conversions of function (as I discuss in *How Brains Think*, conversion and coexistence of functions in the same structure is yet another original insight of Darwin's). And such multi-functionality has some interesting implications for the evolution of new functionality.

You wouldn't think that a new function could spring forth fully formed, as Minerva leaped forth from the head of Jupiter — but it can, thanks to sharing space with an older function. Such bundling of functions constitutes something of a "free lunch." The new function might profit from some additional improvements for efficiency, but its invention per se is not likely to be understood by concentrating on such slow adaptations.

NEW FUNCTIONS USUALLY GET A BIG HEAD START, making part-time use of an organ that, in the past, has been under natural selection for some other, and often quite different, function. Feathers for thermal insulation serving to improve wing aerodynamics is a standard example. Just as the 1940s computers for missile guidance gave a big boost to computers for word processing a few decades later, so brains are particularly capable of conversions of function, improvements in one function stage-setting the emergence of other, seemingly unrelated functions in the off-hours for the original function. The functions might then continue to share the same space, or the space might subdivide into specialists in the two functions.

Because of co-habitation of functions, the labels we use can create some serious blinders. For example, large areas of "language cortex" may be involved with both hand and face movement sequencing — and with analyzing the sequence of sounds you hear. Language cortex isn't exclusively concerned with language. Sensory and motor, hand and face, illustrate the multifunctional reality that brain theories need to cover.

Certainly, just reading the popular press accounts about advances in neuroscience, you'd think that cortex was very specialized, with pigeonholes everywhere: areas for inanimate objects, others for tool concepts, and so on. This recalls Cicero's advice about how to remember new names, which stressed imagining each new person in a different location, such as a room within a large mansion (offering similar advice thirteen centuries later, Thomas Aquinas suggested niches in a cathedral). But, however convenient it may be initially to think of the brain as a *tabula rasa*, with empty pigeonholes at birth waiting to be filled up with a lifetime of memories and acquired skills, few neuroscientists think that it really works that way. Nevertheless, we happily analyze whatever specialties we can find — and, by the functional names we give the area, often blind ourselves to considering additional coexisting functions.

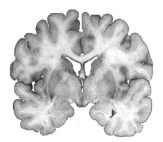

In the experiments of generations of neurophysiologists, individual cortical neurons have often responded to several sensory modalities. Neuroanatomists know that everything is connected to everything (if not directly, then within only several removes). Where they exist, specializations are surely not exclusive, probably in much the same sense that an underutilized neurosurgeon could on occasion help out by doing routine life-insurance physicals in a general medical practice.

SO THE SPECIALIZED-ROOM ANALOGIES won't do, in the long run, however useful they may be for analyzing early stages of perception. I'm going to introduce multifunctionality via some fanciful allusions to the various fields and alcoves within a large public park. Grassy parks such as London's Hampstead Heath are nice, but I have been intrigued with the grassless parks in some cities of Europe, where fine brown gravel walkways cover everything that isn't fenced off.

The park fences are probably due to another tragedy of the commons, I thought, a consequence of the increasing population density inside cities. With more people over the centuries but even less parkland, the open space becomes overused. And then come the fences.

Public spaces such as communal pasture lands have some drawbacks that fencing may avoid, such as overgrazing (where the consequences accrue to the owner of the fenced area, rather than being spread out over everyone who shares the commons). That might, I thought, be one advantage of the departmentalization of the cortex, all those Brodmann Areas. Multifunctional areas of cerebral cortex may, of course, have all the problems associated with a commons — and the tragedies thereof.

Indeed, I observed from a park bench in the center of Paris, some of the graveled areas are flattened so evenly that — well, you don't suppose that the workers have been preparing the surface for the next obvious step?

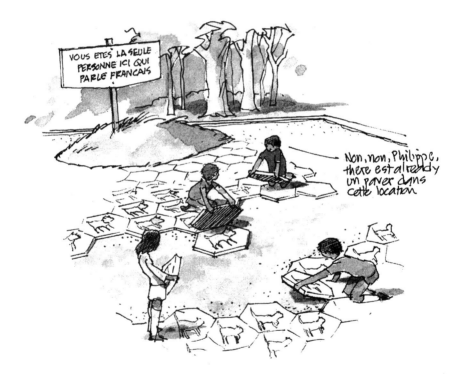

IN MY PARK BENCH REVERIE, the surface was smoothed for exactly that reason. The park officials explain that these aren't permanent tiles that the schoolchildren are laying and repositioning — they're merely *temporary* pavers. (Under the influence of the Greek and Roman bathhouse floors, I originally called them tiles

— but my architect-illustrator gently informed me that tiles implied mortar, that perhaps I had intended to speak of the precast concrete pavers used by homeowners for degrassing the patio?)

The schoolchildren who play in the park will first create a hexagonal mold, its bottom carved into a mascot design. Then they'll pour and lay as many of them as they can, design side up. Some areas will have a standard cat design, and then you might walk across some gravel again until encountering another honeycombed area, each paver having the dog design favored by another group of paver-layers. Since they're all hexagonal in shape, they're easy for the children to lay without exercising any judgment, a nice algorithmic process. A robot could do it.

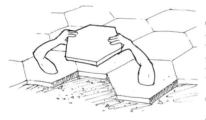

Perhaps, I thought, we could even dispense with the paver-layers and imagine a pair of pavers as sometimes cloning a third with the same characteristic decoration, inserting it into any adjacent unpaved space.

What, you wonder, will happen when the army of cat pavers comes face to face (well, edge to edge) with the dog ones? Will dog pavers replace cat pavers and start taking over the cat territory? Is the size of the dog territory important for some reason? Now, if these were the hexagonal mosaics predicted for cerebral cortex, someone would surely suggest that they have to all fire in synchrony, binding them together so that they will be noticed by an observer on high. I'd prefer to suggest (just wait for chapter 8) that there's a critical number needed before they're likely to communicate effectively with the motor centers of the brain.

Indeed (aren't reveries fun?), leaving aside the cartesian theater fallacy for the moment, what might you see from an aerial photo of this park? Probably lots of alcoves (thanks to those barriers known as foliage) opening off the central spaces, though the extent of the alcoves will be obscured by the overhanging tree branches, as will some of the paths between them (that's one advantage of a map over an aerial photo — and shows why an abstract schema can improve on a "rich mental image").

Up close, of course, there are many things going on simultaneously in this park: wandering around it might reveal country dancing in one alcove, children listening to a storyteller in another alcove, occasionally an alcove with some specialized facilities such as chess tables or a few charcoal grills. Though not suitable for the dancers, such specialized facilities could still be used by

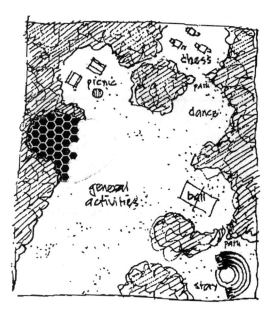

the storyteller. Various paver designs might get started in one alcove or another, with themes reflecting the activities in progress, and then clone their way outward into more general-purpose open spaces, the ones where soccer games alternate with rock concerts and frisbee tag.

I'VE LONG THOUGHT THAT COPYING COMPETITIONS, rather like the paving of that park, must be the way in which my premotor cortex goes about deciding between various alternative actions as I make up my mind. Thumb-up, a precision grip, and pointing might be the contending possibilities. A hexagonal movement schema is, in principle, no different than a sensory one. To an observing neurophysiologist, both would likely be as incomprehensible in appearance as a bar code on a grocery shelf.

Perhaps there is some minimum plurality needed to get the action underway. Perhaps it takes a certain amount of coherent cortical output, enough hexagons worth of movement schemas

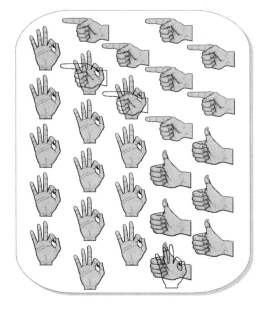

Deciding to act might be a matter of cloning movement commands. Movement might not be initiated until one dominates.

A competition for cortical territory might occur as overlapping patterns are converted into one or the other, depending in part on fading resonances from earlier occupations.

singing in sync as a chorus, in order to persuade the subcortical centers to get their act together.

I expect that for well-learned "cortical reflexes," as when I quickly wave at a friend driving past, the decision making is much simpler. But when there is time for indecision, and where there are various possible actions contending, a copying competition is a nice mechanism for gating thought into action, one solution to the problem of how billions of neurons can make up their collective mind. Perhaps it's a matter of whose song can recruit the largest chorus, and not a manner of annexing all the competing territories — rather as in hegemony, where one nation may dominate the political agendas of a region without actual territorial conquest.

WE HAVE ALREADY IDENTIFIED the first two darwinian essentials, and now we have a candidate for a work space. It's just an analogy so far, but soon it will be fleshed out as like a dynamically changing patchwork quilt of differing hexagonal territories. What about variations on the cloned pattern, ways of making a new individual, one that might clone a new patch and compete with its parent pattern?

There is clearly the possibility of the aforementioned "error correction" preventing any variations on an established pattern, once a given hexagon is surrounded by like-minded ones for crystallization tendencies to assert themselves. But on the edges of a paver area, bordering an unorganized area, a hexagon may only have three or four neighbors. Furthermore, some geometric arrangements of barriers allow only two neighbors to an unorganized hexagon. It is on such frontiers that we should first look for variant patterns, not within the "continents."

Most simply, a hexagonal variant could be caused by the failure of one or more of the triangular arrays to clone new nodes. The spatiotemporal melody within the hexagon would be missing a note, in the manner of a piano with a dead key. This "loss of detail" might mean the dropout of one attribute, such as color, but not necessarily. When we say *yellow* or *horizontal*, we are only emphasizing the most easily investigated attribute of our "feature detector" (itself a convenient fiction). Many interneurons are multisensory and so a given triangular array need not represent a modality that is orthogonal to all other attributes.

A second type of variant would be when new triangular arrays join the collection. The most likely way for this to happen is when two different hexagonal mosaic patterns collide and a "no-man's-land" forms where the two spatiotemporal patterns superimpose (or perhaps they partially inhibit one another, in the clash of incompatible spatiotemporal melodies). There are two aspects of such a no-mans-

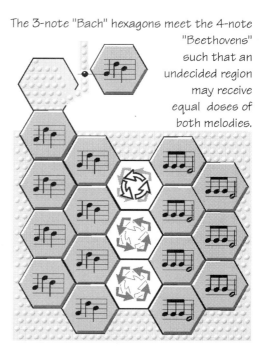

The 3-note "Bach" hexagons meet the 4-note "Beethovens" such that an undecided region may receive equal doses of both melodies.

land: variant patterns and whether the border moves as one tiling replaces another (to be treated in the next chapter, after we examine resonances).

AN EVOLUTIONARY work space is not usually a continent but rather a much smaller region, such as an island or isolated valley or hilltop. Patchy distribution of essential resources can create sub-populations, if migration across the resourceless gaps is infrequent. I'll develop the idea further in *Act II*, but a work space implies more than a blackboard; it's also a region where a sub-population can go extinct, and thereby create an empty niche.

So, too, the relevant cortical work space for cloning competitions is unlikely to be the whole neocortex. The change in the metric associated with the gaps (and the basal dendritic spreads) between adjacent cortical areas may ensure that cloning remains within one Brodmann Area (though the U-fibers of the better-known corticocortical connections might still manage to produce clones, as I will show in chapter 8). Patchy excitatory drive may create even smaller work spaces, as might waves of inhibition.

Much more can (and will) be said about the generation of variants and the size of work spaces, but it will be useful to first consider some cortical possibilities for that fifth essential, the multifaceted environment, now that we have identified the pattern, how it copies, how it might vary, and the limited territory in which it might compete.

The difference between the amoeba and Einstein is that, although both make use of the method of trial and error or elimination, the amoeba dislikes erring while Einstein is intrigued by it: he consciously searches for his errors in the hope of learning by their discovery and elimination.

KARL POPPER, 1979

Intelligent variations require an explanation for how these variations or hypotheses came to be wise-in-advance. That most hypotheses are wise, I have no doubt. As such, they reflect already achieved knowledge or, at very least, wise restrictions on the search space. Such wisdom does not, however, explain further advances in knowledge. That hypotheses, even if not wise, are far from random, I agree. But wise or stupid, restraints on the search space do not explain novel solutions.

DONALD T. CAMPBELL, 1990

A Brief Guide to the Illustrations

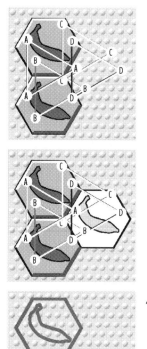

Reality (four or more sets of triangular arrays) is usually too complicated to illustrate, so hexagons are substituted in most illustrations.

A complete active set of triangular arrays for *Banana*, sustained by a basin of attraction in the underlying connectivity, is represented by an icon on a raised hexagon.

A complete active set, merely sustained by recruitment copying from neighboring hexagons, is represented by the flat hexagons with an icon.

A basin of attraction in the underlying connectivity, without an active set manifesting it, is represented by the unfilled icon and hexagon.

If the connectivity changes are fading with time (synaptic depression or reduced facilitation), it is represented by a more ghostly icon.

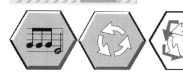

As above, but with reminders that there is a spatiotemporal pattern underlying the hexagon.

5

Resonating with Your Chaotic Memories

[Does memory consist] of the traces of things registered in the mind? What can be the traces of words, of actual objects, what further could be the enormous space adequate to the representation of such a mass of material?

CICERO

Some people do not become thinkers simply because their memories are too good.

FRIEDRICH WILHELM NIETZSCHE

We have to change truth a little in order to remember it.

GEORGE SANTAYANA

ENVIRONMENT IS THAT FIFTH ESSENTIAL for a full-fledged darwinian process. Environments aren't just one thing, though we often speak of them as having one key feature that dominates all others; for example, as if it were simple efficiency at cracking open difficult seeds that makes the difference between the less successful and the more successful finches in the Galapagos, at least during a drought. But typical environments are multifaceted — mental environments ought to be particularly variegated — and they fluctuate widely over a lifetime.

From the standpoint of a darwinian process operating in neocortex, the environment ought to include such things as physiological state, sensory inputs from the outside environment, and memories of earlier ones from an inner environment. In each cortical area, physiological state ought to include the relative ratios of those four major neuromodulators (acetylcholine, serotonin, norepinephrine, and dopamine) arriving from subcortical sites, plus all the peptide neuromodulators. Also, preparedness for action (those holds on movements that might be arriving from prefrontal cortex, those agendas being monitored from orbital frontal) creates behavioral "sets." Thalamus is particularly influential at "activating the EEG" in small regions of neocortex, surely an aspect of selective attention that forms part of the environment for a darwinian process. All of these factors will impinge on the ability of a cortical area to sustain a spatiotemporal pattern, to clone new territory, and to resurrect a spatiotemporal pattern that has fallen silent.

A major part of our environment, however, is a memorized one, and the psychology of memory suggests that it is far more unreliable than is usually thought. Sensory inputs are, by the time they reach the areas of cortex involved with working memory, filtered by perceptual processes. Furthermore, the sensations are averaged over some time past. We don't see the jittery visual field that our eye movements suggest we ought to be seeing; instead we see a stable *model* of that visual world, complete with some of the mistakes we call illusions and hallucinations.

A memory recall, to a psychologist or neurophysiologist, is an even more artificial construction because it isn't anchored by current sensory input. Recalls are created on the fly, sometimes differently on successive occasions, and are potentially tainted by injections from one's imagination. At times, reality becomes suspect because the validity of your memories are called into question. Studies of eyewitnesses to staged mishaps have long suggested that even those eyewitnesses who initially recall the cars, people, and sequence of events correctly can, after a few weeks, get them scrambled up — and not realize it.

THE MEMORIZED ENVIRONMENT is surely the biggest problem we face as we try to make sense of the setting for a darwinian shaping-up process. All the other contributors are potentially active patterns of cell firings or their immediate aftermath.

Environments memorized some time ago surely involve passive spatial-only patterns.

If a hexagon's activity is the relevant spatiotemporal pattern, what is the corresponding spatial-only pattern that can recreate it? It is presumably the synaptic connectivity within the hexagon (in actuality, within a minimum of two adjacent hexagons but, most of the time, likely spanning dozens).

In any one hexagon of cortex, we can distinguish between internally generated spatiotemporal patterns and imposed ones (such as those that are due to recruitment from neighboring hexagons). It's the same distinction as in learning a new dance step, where traditional locomotion spatiotemporal patterns get in the way of copying the instructions from the caller. It's not an either-or situation: each hexagon's connectivity can either aid or hinder an imposed melody via resonance phenomena.

Resonance is what makes Puget Sound (misnamed; it's really a long bay) have a multistory tidal range, while the nearby Pacific Ocean seacoast has only about one-third the range — merely up to the first floor windows, as it were. The time that it takes seawater to slosh back and forth in the bay is similar to the tidal period, and so the amplitude builds up, much like gently pushing a child on a swing at the pendulum's characteristic rate.

Another classic example is the washboarded road, whose bumps and ruts interact with the spatiotemporal bouncing pattern of the moving vehicle. There may be some speed at which the vehicle's tires and springs resonate with the bumps. Increase or decrease your speed by 30 percent and you will probably escape the jarring ride — unless, of course, too many other drivers have tried the same trick and thus created a secondary set of bumps for your new speed. 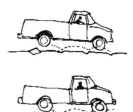 The bumps are created, after all, by bouncing vehicles. Connectivities are the bumps and ruts of the brain; indeed, they are created in part by carving — removing pre-existing connections — and in part by building up other connections.

There isn't a one-to-one mapping between spatial-only and spatiotemporal patterns within the nervous system in the manner of a phonograph recording or sheet music. A given long-term connectivity surely supports many distinct spatiotemporal patterns. In the spinal cord, for example, a given connectivity supports a half-dozen gaits of locomotion, each a distinct spatio-temporal pattern involving many muscles and the relative times of their activation. It is presumably the initial conditions that determine which pattern is elicited from the connectivity.

One aspect of initial conditions is that ghostly blackboard, the fading facilitation of synapses that was caused by earlier activity in the hexagon. Another aspect is the pitter-patter of inputs from thalamus and elsewhere; inputs that are not strong enough to initiate impulses can nonetheless bias the hexagon's resonances. There are also those neuromodulators impinging diffusely on neo-cortex from subcortical areas; likely the relative activity in these systems enhances or masks characteristic resonances. Somewhat more specific inputs from amygdala or thalamus may "shift attention" in a similar way.

CHAOTIC ATTRACTORS ARE A MORE GENERAL WAY of thinking about resonance. There's a fuller discussion of chaos in the Glossary, but the simplest attractors are the *point attractors*, such as the rest state at the bottom of the pendulum's damped swing. The clocklike

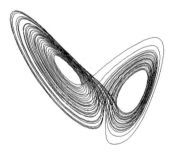

limit-cycle attractors are familiar from the relaxation oscillators that flush and refill reservoirs; there's one that causes the neuron to fire rhythmically on occasion. Bursting cells may have a *quasiperiodic attractor* but, in Walter Freeman's words, "if a system flutters like a butterfly, it may have a chaotic attractor."

Chaotic behavior (in the mathematical sense of the word) looks random. The aperiodic appearance of the waking EEG is one example; physiological tremor is another. Chaos is a pattern difficult to predict because it isn't recursive. But chaos, like mixing with a kitchen egg beater, isn't noise; it is still produced deterministically by the underlying mechanisms.

In deep sleep, the EEG's chaotic behavior is replaced by limit-cycle rhythmicity; in Parkinsonism, the normal chaotic attractor of physiological tremor is said to be replaced by fixed-point attractors (rigidity) and limit-cycle attractors (rhythmic tremor). If there are two attractors mixed up, the system may loop around one attractor and then switch to the other — and in a manner far more complicated than the familiar example of the compound pendulum. The transition between attractors is effectively a phase transition analogous to solid-liquid-gas transitions. Figure-ground illusions provide an example of how an unchanging stimulus pattern may give rise to several (sometimes alternating) perceptions, even if you fixate on a single point.

If we are comatose or under deep anesthesia, point attractors dominate and we experience rest or rigidity. The hierarchy of mental functions builds up from this lowest level, where very little is working, to the level of deep sleep characterized by slow waves, which are also characteristic of the late "clonic" part of seizures. Above that is a level of functioning such as stupor and dementia, where things aren't working very well but at least aren't stuck in the limit cycle of oscillations. As we switch from walking to jogging to running, we change in and out of the various attractors. When the Necker cube switches back and forth between top-down and bottom-up perspectives, it's presumably because we're switching in and out of lobes of an attractor.

OUR MORE INTELLIGENT MENTAL STATES are sometimes said to flirt around the "edge of chaos." This term is from complexity theory, which envisages an adaptive system that ranges between a rigid order and a more flexible disorder, controlling the degree of permitted disorder. We may range from satisfaction at getting something right (convergent thinking) to blue-sky divergent thinking; in those more creative moments, some of our cortical systems may be poised near the edge of chaos. So, just to abstract the term even further from its everyday connotations, chaos is *controlled* disorder!

"Capture" is another aspect of resonance/attractors that will be useful here: a spatiotemporal pattern that comes close to an attractor's pattern will be altered to conform with that of the attractor. When you feel captured by that washboarded road, it's because you really are being shoehorned into an attractor. This convergence is another way of saying that attractors have a *basin of attraction*, a wide set of starting conditions that all eventually lead into the same attractor cycle.

When we listen to a person speaking or read a page of print, much of what we think we see or hear is supplied from our memory. We overlook misprints, imagining the right letters, though we see the wrong ones; and how little we actually hear, when we listen to speech, we realize when we go to a foreign theatre; for there what troubles us is not so much that we cannot understand what the actors say as that we cannot hear their words. The fact is that we hear quite as little under similar conditions at home, only our mind, being fuller of English verbal associations, supplies the requisite material for comprehension upon a much slighter auditory hint.

WILLIAM JAMES, 1899˙

Thus we have convergence to a quasi-reproducible pattern — and that enables a form of sensory generalization (as I'll discuss in *Act II*, the classic example of generalization is getting a monkey to treat a large triangle the same as a small inverted triangle). Categorical perception is but one example of cognitive phenomena that could be effected by capture, as when we listen to a graded range of speech sounds progressing from /ba/ to /pa/. We hear them not as a changing series but as a monotonous repetition of /ba/ that, suddenly, switches to /pa/ repeating over and over (newborns don't have this problem, lacking capture categories). The reason that many native Japanese speakers confuse the English /l/ and /r/ sounds (as when *rice* comes out as *lice*) is an in-between Japanese phoneme whose well-learned-in-infancy category captures *both* English phonemes. That means that the Japanese speaker cannot hear his mistake in English pronunciation ("But I *did* pronounce it exactly the way that you said!").

According to dynamics the stimulus places the cortex in one of its basins of attraction, and the form of the output is determined by the attractor. The finding that perceptual patterns are created by the sensory cortices implies that the cortical dynamics is nonlinear and chaotic, because neither linear operations nor point and limit cycle attractors can create novel patterns. Having played its role in setting the initial conditions, the sense-dependent activity is washed away, and the perceptual message that is sent on into the forebrain is the construction, not the residue of a filter or a computational algorithm. A requirement for this process of "laundering" is for spatial coherence, which arises from cooperativity over the cortical populations. This process of replacement of sensory inputs by endogenous constructions in perception constitutes the basis of epistemological solipsism in brains.

WALTER J. FREEMAN, 1995

AFTER ALL THIS BACKGROUND on memory, and the loose analogies to chaos and complexity, we can now consider how an unorganized cortical territory is influenced by resonances when a spatiotemporal pattern arrives by lateral cloning. If the cloning pattern resonates with the connectivity, annexation will be easier than if it doesn't. Indeed, perhaps the new region will adopt the rhythm so enthusiastically that the pattern will locally persist, even if the lateral copying that ignited it were to be discontinued.

On the other hand, were the cortex sufficiently excitable that all patterns reliably cloned laterally, resonances would not matter. The local maintenance of the rhythm, however, would then be totally dependent on lateral copying. It would be easily erased, in comparison to resonating regions that kept going when a supply route was temporarily interrupted. The copying-only case is like a group of novice dancers learning a new spatiotemporal pattern by following instructions from a caller (as in square dance); when the caller stops, so do they. But eventually, as the dancers develop their own internal resonances, they can generate the patterns on their own, sans caller.

Locally, graded effects might be important for getting the rhythm started, much as piano keys can be struck softly or vigorously. Once into lateral cloning mode, however, the notes might be as stereotyped as those plucked notes on a harpsichord, more digital than analog — with copying from copies, you probably need a digital code, as shades of grays eventually go to all-or-nothing extremes (much as photocopying the previous photocopy of a photograph will progress to an image with a solarized black-and-white appearance). So our cerebral code is likely to be binary, even though calling it up from scratch may have important analog aspects.

Note that we now have a serious reason for treating the hexagon as more than just a convenient group name for a collection of N points from N triangular arrays. Yes, extension of territory initially involves each triangular array recruiting a new node in the no-mans-land — but resonances mean that some sequences fit into a locally favored melody, and some don't. The favored melody is a property of the hexagon's connectivity, as manifested by the attractors.

MEMORIZING A SPATIOTEMPORAL PATTERN would seem to be a matter of creating a new connectivity, probably in a number of hexagons. Although the usual LTP-to-structural-enhancement model of learning (some synapses are enlarged in the days following LTP) seems to suffice here, remember that we are superimposing some connectivity changes upon a pre-existing cortical connectivity, one that already has some attractors inherent in it.

Tacking on yet another attractor may not always be possible. One reason is that strong local attractors can likely capture the new pattern once lateral copying is discontinued, altering the pattern to the previously stored one, and so the new one is never memorized.

But don't forget the spatial aspect: a successful new spatiotemporal pattern has probably temporarily occupied dozens to hundreds of hexagons. Although some hexagons may capture the new pattern once active cloning discontinues, others may be able to accommodate the permanent connectivity change that would make later recall of the new spatiotemporal pattern possible. This redundancy accords well with Lashley's notion that memory traces are widespread, while still allowing for some expert areas.

While the connectivity change, when successfully made, might eliminate one of the weaker attractors of the pre-existing collection, as I will discuss in chapter 9, a locally lost basin of attraction probably has stronger versions elsewhere. Once cortical "slots" start to fill up, finding a suitable niche for adding a new attractor may require hexagonal mosaics that temporarily annex a lot of cortex (you might need to pay a lot of attention to a new event, in order for it to be recorded). This also means that the new attractor may be scattered, evocable from isolated pockets here and there (one of the surprises of early chaos theory was that basins of attraction could be parcellated), but the scattered nature might make it more difficult to get a critical mass going during recall attempts.

Memory recall is now easier to imagine with such attractor mosaics: the revival of the ingrained spatiotemporal pattern could start from any place in the original annexation territory and, once re-ignited, spread by lateral cloning to annex a somewhat different territory. This is a nice feature because recall need not begin from the very feature detectors (perhaps scattered over some millimeters) that started everything, back during acquisition, before synchronous recruitment extended some triangular arrays. The cloning might even spread back into the original feature detectors, but I can see no reason why this would be necessary for either percepts or concepts. The criterion for successful output may simply be enough active clones of a spatiotemporal pattern to instruct the motor pathways, not activity in a particular neuron set.

As an aside, note that neocortical memory capacity might well be limited. The price of memorizing a new phone number, well enough to recall it tomorrow, might be eliminating a resonance for some other memory — say, the name of your first-grade teacher. Usually, there would be other attractors for that name elsewhere, but eventually you might eliminate the last one because the new attractor's connectivity change will produce a connectivity pattern in those hexagons which can no longer resurrect that characteristic pattern. The remaining connectivity might still resonate with imposed patterns, so you might continue to recognize the name when you heard it, but recall per se will stop working.

The age at which this gain-one-lose-another state of affairs begins is an empirical question. Nothing in the hexagons theory suggests whether it should occur at age 10 or age 80, but the theory does suggest an experimental strategy of looking for a developing gap between recognition and recall of long-term memories.

A SIMPLE SENSORY DECISION now looks rather like that hand movement decision earlier. The cortex would have some resonances for

Active
Pattern

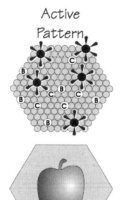

The connectivity that generates the spatiotemporal patterns must be able to produce, for different initial conditions, dozens of active "melodies," just as the spinal cord generates the spatiotemporal patterns for the gaits of locomotion.

Passive
Connectivity

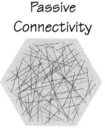

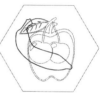

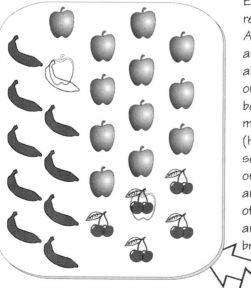

Even when the resonances for *Apple, Banana,* and *Cherry* are all omnipresent, one pattern may be able to clone more successfully (here *Apple* is seen encroaching on both *Banana* and *Cherry*) because of extrinsic biases arriving from other brain regions.

EMOTIONS
DRIVES
SENSES

Banana and *Apple* and *Cherry*; there would be hexagons that resonated to all three, just as the spinal cord circuitry supports multiple gaits of locomotion. Some hexagons might resonate to certain patterns better than others.

Which succeeds in cloning the largest territory, however, will surely depend on both permanent basins of attraction and some temporary ones. For example, hexagons from which the *Apple* spatiotemporal pattern has retreated will likely have some lingering aftereffects; perhaps facilitation and LTP will leave the connectivity in a state more likely to support the reestablishment of *Apple*. Such passive patterns are superimposed on the hexagon's permanent connectivity; they might make it easier (or more difficult) for them to be activated (psychologists love to talk about proactive and retroactive inhibition of memories).

One can also imagine ways to avoid a resonance, simply by using a triangular array on a different slant in the cortex. The very same territory might be associated with other rhythms operating through triangular arrays on some other slant; they, too, could have anchored hexagons in this "alternate universe." This has interesting implications for the multifunctionality of neocortical areas, the conflict between Lashley's equipotentiality and the neurologists' specialized anomias. In particular, one could avoid specialist attractors by using other slants and so achieve a temporary work space.

MANY MEMORY RECALL PHENOMENA seem dependent on recreating a physiological state similar to that at initial presentation, as when things learned under the influence of alcohol are more easily recalled after a few drinks. Some of this might be explained by staging attractors, and some by finding the right slant for the array.

But such enhancement by association is only one instance of a much more general phenomena: that of setup actions (or, as the more extreme versions are known, reconfiguration actions). Neuromodulators such as serotonin and dopamine serve to sculpt particular circuits out of networks by enhancing some connection strengths and reducing others (or shortening and lengthening their actions). Some attractors thus fade into the background and

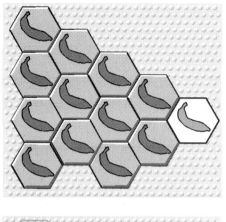

*Basins of Attraction
Can Be Avoided
by Altering Angle
of Active Arrays*
Facilitation and LTP
may leave behind altered
connectivity. These ghostly
images are basins of attraction
overlaid on those of the
permanent connectivity.

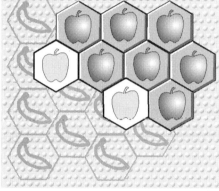

One way of avoiding these
basins of attraction may be
to plate hexagonal mosaics
at a different angle. In this
manner, an adjacent cortical
area could use this one as a
temporary workspace, avoiding
both its permanent specialist
attractors and any fading
ones from earlier occupations
at the usual angle and offset.

others pop out. Fading facilitation from earlier triangular arrays, ones that are no longer active in the sense of maintaining spatiotemporal firing patterns, also can serve a setup function, biasing what attractors are most easily accessed.

Much of the foregoing could be said for schemes other than triangular array extension and the consequent hexagonal mosaics. As Peter Getting said about motor systems, "input may not only *activate* a network but may *configure* it into an appropriate mode to process that input." The entrainment of the triangular arrays, however, has some specific predictions to make about what gets memorized and what doesn't.

As mentioned earlier (p. 32), the NMDA types of postsynaptic receptors for the excitatory neurotransmitter glutamate are especially common in the superficial layers. The connections between our recurrently exciting superficial pyramidal neurons surely utilize NMDAlike properties. What features might NMDA augment?

The NMDA receptor for glutamate also requires the presence of some glycine in order to open up its channel through the neuron's membrane. (Another "duality" is that, in the spinal cord, glycine is an inhibitory neurotransmitter). The channel associated with the NMDA receptor seems to allow both sodium and calcium ions into the neuron. But its most singular "dual" property is that, unlike conventional synaptic channels, the NMDA ion channel is controlled by the binding of the neurotransmitter *and* by the pre-existing 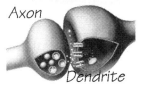 voltage across that membrane. It seems that magnesium ions tend to get stuck in the channel, effectively blocking it, so that even if glutamate binds to the NMDA receptor, no current flows through the ion channel to contribute to an excitatory postsynaptic potential. An EPSP may nonetheless be seen, of course, because non-NMDA channels are also activated by the glutamate, allowing sodium ions in, but the EPSP will not be as large as otherwise. Blocked NMDA channels represent a reserve; there's extra responsiveness available for special occasions requiring emphasis.

Reducing the voltage gradient across the membrane (depolarization), however, tends to pop loose the trapped Mg^{++}. In consequence, the next glutamate that binds to the NMDA receptor will gate a flow of sodium and calcium ions into the parent channel and so raise the internal voltage of the dendrite to make a larger EPSP. The functional consequence of this channel clearing is that the dendrite becomes much more sensitive to the *history* of arrivals.

For example, two impulses arriving a few milliseconds apart sum together nonlinearly. The second hump may be substantially larger than otherwise, thanks to the NMDA channels cleared by the first EPSP. In LTP experiments, a long train of impulses in a given pathway is produced, likely clearing out most of the blocked NMDA channels. The presynaptic terminal also becomes more likely to release glutamate when the next impulse arrives, thanks to some retrograde transmitter from the NMDA postsynaptic response feeding back to the presynaptic terminal.

But an EPSP arriving in another part of the dendrite may be nearly as effective at augmenting the NMDA channel's EPSP; it's the voltage change produced at the NMDA channel's location that is important, not whether that particular channel contributed to the voltage production. This means that near-synchronous inputs (say, within about 10 msec of one another) are far more effective than would otherwise be the case, and that postsynaptic impulses retrogradely invading the dendrites should also unblock some NMDA channels (providing yet another mechanism for "Hebbian synapses"). Absolute synchrony isn't required, as it is simply a matter of how long it takes for another Mg^{++} to get trapped in the ion channel (often tens to hundreds of msec). Well-focused triangular nodes would benefit from a narrower window that could detect conduction-time coincidences (though surround inhibition is also available to shrink and focus the hot spot, once it develops).

Repeated "synchrony" of two inputs, as predicted for the triangular arrays, might be the closest natural situation to the LTP experiments that produce enhancements in synaptic strength of a few hundred percent. Add to this the widespread suspicion that long-lasting changes in synaptic strength are built on a scaffolding provided by LTP changes, and you have one plausible recipe for triangular arrays embedding a new pattern in the connectivity, there to linger for a lifetime.

Although triangular array extensions can presumably occur without NMDA receptors, it seems clear that the NMDA properties could provide a lot of enhancement to recurrent excitation's tendencies to entrain neurons. And NMDA isn't the only enhancer: the apical dendrite (the tall stalk that rises from the cell body toward to cortical surface before branching; see p. 26) seems to have many voltage-sensitive ion channels, including the persistent sodium channels and calcium channels. They allow antecedent depolarizations, in effect, to amplify the currents produced by a subsequent synaptic input. Indeed, more than half the 2X amplification seen at the cell body, from mimicking glutamate synaptic activation a half mm up the apical dendrite, seems to be from such mechanisms, with NMDA-dependent mechanisms under the synapse contributing a similar amount to the overall amplification.

AUTOMATIC GAIN CONTROLS (AGCs) have become familiar from the way that some tape recorders automatically control their loudness. On replay, you hear the background hiss fade out, shortly after someone begins talking, whereupon background voices also become fainter. That is because the recording gain is automatically adjusted downward when, averaged over the last second or two, there has been lots of input.

AGC mechanisms per se have not yet been described in neocortex, though surround inhibition accomplishes somewhat the same thing, as does long-term depression. AGCs would seem useful for avoiding a fog of the characteristic patterns. With all the recurrent excitation in superficial layers of neocortex, there is a great need to keep the system from becoming regenerative. Voltage-sensitive potassium currents help to keep the lid on things, but that's a mechanism limited to inside one neuron, not one that can influence neighbors as well, in the manner of one loud voice turning down the loudness of the background voices in that tape recording.

Association cortex lacks a lot of the spontaneous firing that we see elsewhere in the central nervous system. Sustained firing is usually seen only in the major sensory receiving areas, in response to particularly effective stimuli, or in motor areas during preparation for movement. But while cortical neurons are individually capable of firing rhythmically to sustained synaptic inputs, they usually don't. One survey shows that they're suspiciously nonrhythmic, with intervals between impulses being much more random than we would have expected. Something such as a cortical AGC is presumably limiting the more vigorous rhythmic activity.

From the NMDA properties, we can imagine how a simple, nonspecific AGC might work. After all, the extension of a triangular array contributes to a lot of nonspecific activation of cortical cells. Besides the hot spots where excitatory annuli overlap, there is a much stimulation of nonfocal areas by the other axon branches. Suppose that Mg^{++} was released by activity (or that some diffusing metabolite served to increase intracellular free Mg^{++} levels), so that there was more opportunity to block the NMDA channels that had been cleaned out. This would preferentially reduce the synaptic strengths in those paths. If the magnesium messenger diffused for macrocolumnar distances or the glia did similar work, it might well dampen the impulse activity in the rest of the region, leaving only the more optimally stimulated hot spots as the islands of activity that continue to maintain the raised "sea level."

Inhibitory mechanisms are the usual way of reducing the widespread anatomical funnel to the much smaller physiologically active area, but simple AGCs of this sort might easily help narrow the catchment zone for effective recurrent excitation. The necessity for a little glycine as a co-factor for the usual excitatory neurotransmitter at NMDA receptors would fit well with an AGC that spread a lot of glycine around as a neuromodulator: while suppressing excitability in general, it could conceivably augment NMDA synapses so that their neurons stood out. (Sea level might rise, but the hilltops still above water might be stimulated to grow!) Contrast is everything.

WE NEED TO ABANDON THE STRING QUARTET at this juncture. If my digital-analog analysis is correct, each of the members of that little choral cluster is really a one-note specialist. You will probably have some difficulty imagining a specialized soprano that can only sing a high C, and nothing else. Because the hexagon has on the order of a hundred minicolumns, however, we can refine our musical analogy to a harpsichord keyboard; each singer is really only one key, either sounding briefly or keeping quiet. You get to map the hundred minicolumns to your musical synthesizer keyboard in whatever way sounds most pleasing to your ears, as each has no inherent tonal quality. My analogy is simply a way of translating one pattern into a more familiar one, just as we translate high-pitched dolphin vocalizations into our own auditory range in order to aid our efforts at detecting patterns in the performance.

Theory cannot yet provide much guidance on some critical questions: How many attractors can a hexagon's worth of connectivity support before filling up? How easy is it to overlay another basin of attraction on the existing ones? Or to dislodge an existing attractor? How might "subliminal" inputs to a neocortical area (ones that do not themselves generate impulses, much less triangular arrays) bias the attractors and their approach basins?

Note that the present theory does not aspire to the traditional goal of cortical circuit models, those transformations of sensory input that underlie perception. It aspires, rather, to the more abstract aspects of analogy needed for categories and creativity, able to generate new levels of sophisticated complexity. Nor does this theory have much to say about what determines the temporal aspect of spatiotemporal patterning — in the manner, say, of the coincidence cascades, postulated by Moshe Abeles, or the structuring role of the EEG "carriers" that may aid the widespread establishment of synchrony, emphasized by Peter König, Wolf Singer, and Andras Engel. My theory can, fortunately, say a lot more about some of the overall spatial dynamics, the possible neocortical equivalents of boom and bust.

The more difficult and novel the problem, the greater is likely to be the amount of trial and error required to find a solution. At the same time, the trial and error is not completely random or blind; it is, in fact, rather highly selective. The new expressions that are obtained by transforming given ones are examined to see whether they represent progress toward the goal. Indications of progress spur further search in the same direction; lack of progress signals the abandonment of a line of search. Problem solving requires selective trial and error.

HERBERT A. SIMON, 1969

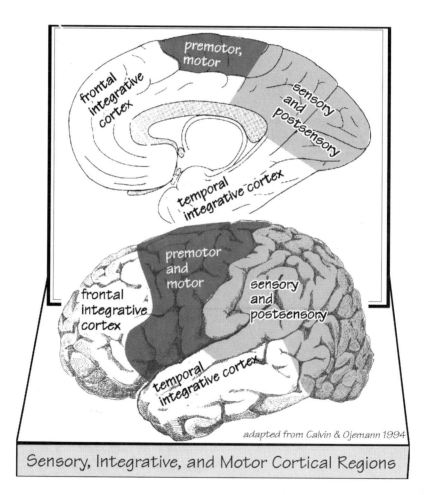

adapted from Calvin & Ojemann 1994

Sensory, Integrative, and Motor Cortical Regions

6

Partitioning the Playfield

[The genes vs. bodies] genotype-phenotype duality of the living organism is the reason why it is not sufficient in biology to search for a single cause in the study of a phenomenon, as is often sufficient in the physical sciences.

ERNST MAYR, 1988

EBB'S DUAL TRACE MEMORY had long seemed to me to constitute a possible analog to the genes versus bodies distinction. Throughout the 1980s, I kept thinking about spatial-only long-term memory traces and contrasting them with spatiotemporal patterns for active memory (p. 17), hoping to see an analogy to genes somewhere.

As it turns out, nothing in my hexagons theory is analogous to the "germ line," the genes that are unaffected by feedback from the body (but whose chances of being successfully copied are dependent on the body). The biological two-levels tradition was, however, quite influential in how I came to see Hebb's dual-trace-memory problem. Getting from there to here has depended on quite a few additional developments in science.

John Z. Young kicked off the neural round of selectionist thinking with his 1964 book, *A Model of the Brain*, where he discussed tuning up the nervous system by weakening synapses. Richard Dawkins touched on the same theme in 1971, extending it to selective cell death; outside of prenatal development, neuronal death is not currently considered an important candidate. Dawkins's real contribution has turned out to be on the copying side, not the selection side, of mental darwinism. In his 1976 book, *The Selfish Gene*, he extended the notion of copying genes to copying memes (cultural entities such as words and tunes). It took awhile before anyone realized its implications for copying inside a single brain.

Jean-Pierre Changeux's selective stabilization of developing synapses confirmed me in thinking that selecting among the possibilities, and letting self-organization adjust the connection strengths, made far more sense of the known neurobiology than other approaches. Then Gerald Edelman convinced me in the summer of 1977 that a selectionist approach to higher brain functions could be made from the level of pathways and synapses. It was a very liberating view, helping me make sense out of the fuzzy wiring of the brain, the extensive variability between individuals (such as a three-fold range in size of primary visual cortex among adults), and all of those "silent" synapses that we were discovering. Edelman emphasized that to the newborn animal, the world was an unlabeled place and that adaptive mechanisms in the brain had to partition the objects and events of the individual's experience.

When chaos theory came along (which, for me, is dated to Otto Rössler's famous paper of 1983), it started to become evident how basins of attraction lived in the connectivity. When complexity theory and artificial life came along on its heels, the possibilities of getting to the bottom of Hebb's dual-trace memory seemed promising. Then in 1988, I spent more than two months digesting Edelman's *Neural Darwinism*, thanks to a request from *Science* to write a book review that explained it all.

I SAID THAT *NEURAL DARWINISM* was essential reading (and it still is) for anyone interested in brains and development, though it is an unnecessarily difficult book. What I didn't see, in my reading of Edelman, was any role for the repeated copying of active spatiotemporal patterns, particularly as a prelude to the selection step. He seemed to have an intriguing analogy to evolutionary biology, but with the reproducing populations left out. The nature of analogies, of course, is that you always leave something out; the issue is whether what's left out is central to the theme, potentially leaving you confused by a hollow or crippled analogy.

Even if you are adding new synapses all the time, selection by itself is merely a carving process and, although it sometimes introduces interesting patterns, it has none of the power of the full darwinian process with its six essentials and various catalysts. Edelman's "reentry," in the sense of repeated interactions with other regions providing "differential amplification of particular variants in a population," didn't carry the connotation of repeatedly copying a spatiotemporal pattern, such as an ephemeral "fabric" with many cloned repeats of the unit spatio-temporal "swatch."

Most such confusions of darwinian concepts did not detract from the power of Edelman's analysis. But some do, as when he says, "[This] is a population theory, that is, it claims that brains operate by selection upon variance at several levels. Such a process leads to differential modification of synapses and the selection of particular neuronal groups on the basis of individual experience in an open-ended world or environment." All true, except something of a non sequitur. Populations — in ecology and evolutionary biology, and even in immunology — usually involve lots of individuals somehow making near copies of themselves, all present at the same time, interacting with one another and with the environment.

I have a difficult time identifying either an individual unit or a copying mechanism in Edelman's lots-of-neurons notion of a "population." His differential amplification via re-entrant loops, although undoubtedly an important process, doesn't really involve a population in the way the word is used elsewhere in biology. Francis Crick's famous quip, that *Neural Darwinism* ought to be called "neural Edelmanism" instead, is supposed to remind us not to conflate selectionist carving with the darwinian algorithm, the bootstrapping process that makes quality products from crude beginnings.

But even if Edelman's selectionism and populations do not encompass the full-fledged darwinian process (the six essentials and those "catalysts," p.21), his term "neural darwinism" did correspond to the popular notion of darwinism as a carving process, a notion shared by many scientists. If we are to blame anyone for the frequent confusion of selectionism with the full darwinian process, we would have to start with Charles Darwin himself, who named his theory for only one aspect of the six-part process: natural selection.

TRULY DARWINIAN EVOLUTION requires populations of nearly identical individuals, with enough variation for selection to skew reproduction and enough climate fluctuations to pump the process. Could you get darwinian shaping merely from a loop between two cortical maps, the back-and-forth interactions between them serving to adjust both of them? That's Edelman's going-beyond-selectionism idea, though his terminology often has to be translated for the uninitiated.

The road to wisdom?
Well, it's plain and simple to express:
Err and err and err again
but less and less and less.

PIET HEIN

Edelman, quite properly, doesn't like the control systems connotations of "feedback" (technically speaking, there's a standard being compared to an erroneous version that needs correcting). But instead of using "loops" to avoid the error connotation, he used the term "reentry" — though not especially

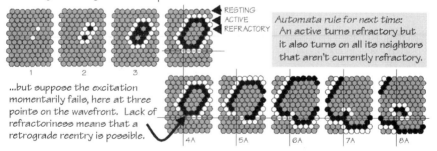

Exciting the neighbors can produce a wavefront...

RESTING
ACTIVE
REFRACTORY

Automata rule for next time: An active turns refractory but it also turns on all its neighbors that aren't currently refractory.

...but suppose the excitation momentarily fails, here at three points on the wavefront. Lack of refractoriness means that a retrograde reentry is possible.

with the "sneaking behind the lines" connotation that the term has acquired in automata theory and cardiac physiology, thus adding to the confusion.

I can imagine Edelman's back and forth adjustment process between maps serving to implement a a shaping-up process, just as subsequent versions of a marked-up manuscript show improvement. Indeed, the analogy to the editorial process suggests a useful (though somewhat shopworn) name: *revisionism*. It is surely slower, less amenable to the traditional darwinian multiple-species competitions, and less algorithmic than proper darwinism; most of the six essentials are hard to identify. However appropriate it may be for the days-to-years time scale that Edelman discusses, shaping up quality in milliseconds-to-minutes may require population-based darwinism, all the six essentials, most of the known catalysts, and perhaps even some unique-to-the-brain shortcuts based on them as well — just to keep us speedy enough to avoid *avoir l'esprit de l'escalier.*

I like the Edelmanian interacting maps for other applications, one of the most important of which is embedding one-trial episodic memories into neocortical connectivity. The more usual skill-acquisition memories that involve many repeated trials have repeated opportunities to embed a new attractor. One-trial learning does exist, but episodic memories are the first to go if memory malfunctions from head injuries, aging, or simply loss of sleep (we tend to guess wrong, or confabulate, rather than realize that we don't know). Eyewitness memories are notoriously unreliable — indeed, they are malleable, with subsequent errors in recall becoming memories themselves, more accessible than the truth.

A rehearsal process during the consolidation of an episodic memory, to imitate repeated trials, is one obvious possibility. I like to think of hippocampus (actually entorhinal cortex, to which hippocampus is a subprocessorlike appendage) triggering the neocortex with the first few notes of the melody, perhaps during sleep or other idle periods, and the cortex responding with the whole line of "music" (or perhaps entorhinal sending the short "message digest" and the neocortex elaborating it into the full "text" of the episode).

But rehearsal isn't cloning either, not any more than reentry is.

CLONING WAS FINALLY ON MY MIND again by 1991. It wasn't the first time. A decade earlier, I'd hypothesized cloning of cortical spatiotemporal patterns as a way of curing timing jitter, getting around the inherent noise of the neuron via an emergent property of a common neural circuit. I'd even taken my original notion of cloning movement commands and extended it to the hyperacuity problem in sensation. No thanks to me, *clone* had also become an everyday word in the 1980s. This time around, I was looking for cortical circuitry that could do the cloning job.

In November 1991, while talking to my old friend Jennifer S. Lund at the neuroscience meetings in New Orleans, things clicked. She was explaining her monkey visual cortex poster to me when I asked about the intrinsic horizontal connection's regularity that she mentioned in passing. Oh yes, Jenny said, that's nothing new, we saw it about ten years ago in the cortex of the tree shrew. Earlier I'd been talking about synchronization of relaxation oscillators with some experts, finding out that entrainment was even more profound than I'd thought from my earlier work (it could be hard to *avoid*, given slight excitatory coupling). All of what has become chapter 2 began to hang together. On the airplane that night, and in a standing-room-only waiting room in the Miami airport en route to visiting my wife's parents, I sketched out what in subsequent months became the hexagons theory. It probably helped that my in-law's apartment had a hexagonal tile floor. I gave my first public lectures on the theory about two months later, to the Seattle neurophysiologists and to the Boston cognitive science community.

I promptly discovered that I would need to explain niches and population thinking while I was at it.

CONCEPTS FROM EVOLUTIONARY BIOLOGY and its "population thinking" are not well known among nervous system researchers or those who would mimic the brain via inventing artificial intelligences. I'd only learned about them myself in the 1980s when I'd volunteered to teach biology to honors-program undergraduates (I'd somehow missed taking introductory biology myself, so I'd had the problem of staying ahead of my bright students in some areas of biology). Population biology has some useful concepts to remember when venturing into the spatio-temporal aspects of a neocortical darwinism, as do the newer concepts of evolutionarily stable strategies, the applications of game theory to interacting populations.

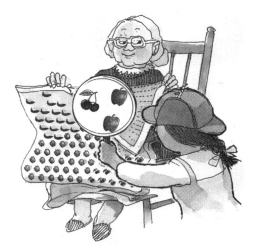

In some sense, it suffices to imagine a dynamically reforming patchwork quilt, each patch's fabric pattern having lots of triangular arrays that, on closer inspection of swatches, constitute cloning hexagons. But population thinking requires more. It involves learning how to phrase the questions in population terms, so as to see both the individual and the population in the manner of seeing both the tree and the forest.

There are, for example, barriers to populations such as mountains, deserts, and large bodies of water. They partition the playfield into parcels (they *parcellate* it), creating regionally isolated subpopulations (*demes*) that don't often interbreed. Most importantly, barriers have gaps that function as gateways. Hikers call them *passes* while mariners call them *passages*, which is perhaps a better term for our mostly flat paving-the-park analogy. The neocortical version of a gateway is what encourages variant spatiotemporal patterns to form individuals that differ slightly from the clones that serve as their parents.

ESCAPING ERROR CORRECTION involves keeping most of the six neighbors to a hexagon (p. 41) from ganging up on the variant. The simplest way to accomplish this is with patchy unresponsive areas, where triangular arrays are unable to recruit followers.

Lack of excitation, the usual tendency of a lot of activity to produce surround inhibition a la Békésy and Hartline (and the recurrent connections of the layer 5-6 pyramidal neurons are a candidate), preoccupation with other activities — all could serve as a *barrier* that limited the spread of a mosaic. In paving-the-park, it would correspond to the mindless paver-layers running into a curb — or perhaps a ridge line thrown up by an enterprising gopher enlarging an underground tunnel.

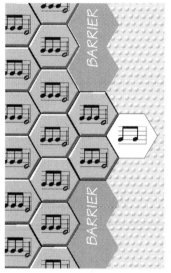

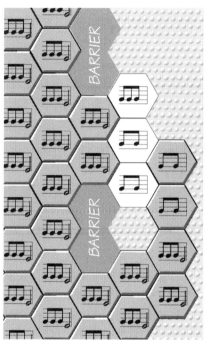

A BARRIER will not support triangular array extension. The reasons might be anatomical (lack of standard-length axon segments) or temporary (insufficient background excitation).

A GATEWAY is an excitable gap in the barrier, about two hexagons wide, where the loss of error correcting neighbors can permit variants to arise.

If two copies of the same variant get started, this novel spatiotemporal pattern may be able to clone. If it is closer to a basin of attraction, it may successfully compete for territory with the parent pattern.

Wide gateways, like wide slits in the physicists's particle-wave experiments, aren't very interesting. Narrow ones, about the width of the local "0.5 mm" metric, stop annexation altogether. It takes activity in two *adjacent* hexagons to clone a third: just recall that lab coat campaign button that reads *Don't Clone Alone!* But gateway widths between two and three times the metric provide a way to escape error correction.

Just through the gateway, triangular array nodes are only subject to the two nodes occupying the gateway. For some of the multiple triangular arrays that constitute the hexagon's spatio-temporal pattern, a failure to recruit might occur. Or a neuron will instead be recruited off to one side of the equilateral triangle, simply because of imprecise anatomy. It is perhaps only with six surrounding neighbors that the nodes are forced into the proper equilateral triangles, just as crystals may be imperfect near their natural edges.

On the far side of the gateway, the imperfect hexagon's triangular arrays will still be able to take part in producing another hexagon, acting in combination with one of the perfect hexagons in the narrow passage. If the imperfect pattern is again created, then there are two imperfect hexagons side by side, the essential setup for cloning a lot more of them.

Although a sexually reproducing species can colonize a new island via just one pregnant female, the asexual cortical hexagons seem to require two to tango.

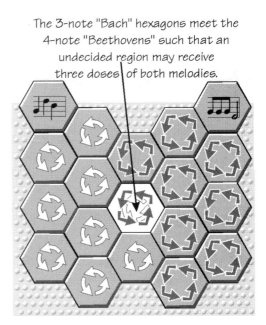

The 3-note "Bach" hexagons meet the 4-note "Beethovens" such that an undecided region may receive three doses of both melodies.

COMPETITION with the parent pattern seems quite likely, particularly if the parent pattern simply does an end run around the barrier. Soon the variants will be contending for the no-mans-land (p. 59) that separates them from the parent clones.

Thanks to concepts such as basins of attraction and how they might be biased by noncloning long-distance inputs, we can imagine why one pattern might succeed better than another in annexing no-mans-land. Indeed, we can ask about how this battlefront moves and stabilizes by considering a three-array spatiotemporal pattern called *Bach* meeting up with a four-array pattern such as *Beethoven*.

Suppose that the undecided territory has shrunken to only one unfilled tile's worth, and that it has three Bach neighbors trying to recruit it via annexing nodes in its three triangular arrays. But it also has the three Beethoven neighbors, also trying to recruit the four corresponding nodes of their arrays. The underlying resonances ought to make the difference in which wins: it's the equivalent of a *memorized* environment biasing a darwinian copying competition. (They might merely superimpose, a topic I'll save for *Act II*.)

Boundaries seem more likely to form along an angle, however, such that all the hexagons on the border have four similar inputs but only two of the other pattern. Although a well-resonating pattern on the two-side might nonetheless invade the territory of a less resonant pattern, four-to-two probably creates a temporary stability in the midst of change.

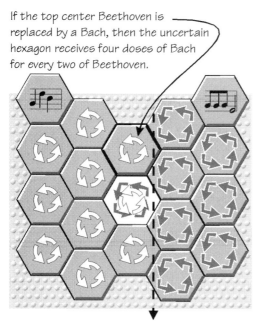

If the top center Beethoven is replaced by a Bach, then the uncertain hexagon receives four doses of Bach for every two of Beethoven.

A 4-by-2 boundary ought to be a more stable one than a 3-by-3 arrangement.

AMBIGUOUS PERCEPTIONS provide a useful example of how copying competitions could perform a common mental task. When overlearned objects are sensed, there is likely no need for a copying competition to decide the issue: they probably immediately pop through to an appropriate attractor and "early decision" obviates the need for prolonged copying. But a lot of what we see is ambiguous, at least temporarily.

Suppose that you see an object go whizzing past, which then disappears beneath something. You can't take a closer look. But what was it? It was seemingly roundish, about the size of many kinds of balls and fruit. How do you guess what it was? Perhaps you use the cortical equivalent of the immune response.

In terms of a cortical darwinian competition, the first task is to take the spatiotemporal pattern of the sensory input, good old "?" (hereafter called *unknown*), and make a territory of clones in a region of cortex that we might call the sensory buffer. A barrier with a gateway will then allow variants to be made on this original group of triangular arrays. A series of additional short end-runable barriers with gateways (not shown) can allow further variants from the original (the distorted *?* in the figure). Finally one of the variant spatio-temporal patterns gets close enough to the *lemon* attractor to be captured by it: a few *lemon* clones form up in one part of the territory. About the same time, the *baseball* attractor has been

Darwin Machine handles ambiguity, finding candidates, and making decision

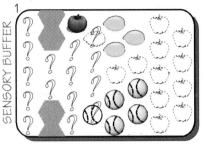

Inexcitable barrier prevents error correction, allows gateway variants.

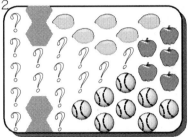

Three candidates have been found via variants being captured by an attractor.

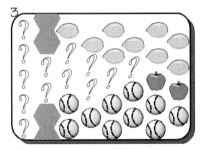

Competition ensues, skewed by extrinsic biases and fading traces.

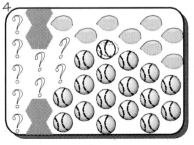

Critical mass: "It was a baseball!"

similarly activated by a different variant, aided by the fact that you're currently at a picnic (*baseball* and *picnic* perhaps have an association in your brain). In a third part of the cortical territory for handling ambiguous visual objects, *apple* has been fired up.

It's possible to simply have a stalemate between *unknown* and the three candidates. But background conditions change much more quickly than the weather — and so *lemon* takes over much of *apple* territory. Finally, *baseball* not only converts many of the remaining *unknown* variants but also the *apple* territory. Because having a number of clones in sync is a good way for long corticocortical paths to get the attention of premotor and language cortex (to be discussed in chapter 8), we get the decision: "It was a baseball."

It's a very simple-minded example of how a perceptual task could get some help from a darwinian cloning competition when there's too much ambiguity for a quick decision. First, variants are spawned. Second, attractors capture some variants and thus create standard spatiotemporal patterns for vocabulary items. Third, a cloning competition ensues, aided by some fluctuations in background excitability. Finally, a decision occurs when there are enough of one type singing in a chorus.

JUST AS CLIMATE FLUCTUATIONS speed up biological evolution, so cortical excitability fluctuations might speed up hexagonal competitions. Some areas will be converted from prepared-for-pavers into barriers that partition the playfield.

A raised threshold in a region (another way of saying reduced excitability or increased inhibition) can be envisaged as humps thrown up by that enterprising gopher. It's not really a fence, in the sense of enclosure, but simply the equivalent of underbrush that's easier to go around than through. Neither does it necessarily partition anything (think instead of those alcoves that open out into the more general-purpose parts of the park, p.56).

> The capacity to blunder slightly is the real marvel of DNA. Without this special attribute, we would still be anaerobic bacteria and there would be no music.
>
> LEWIS THOMAS, 1979

Barriers help fragment reproducing populations so that they can go their own way, unconstrained by interactions with the other demes or the main population itself. The second consequence is, of course, that the narrower gaps between barriers permit reproduction of hexagonal spatiotemporal firing patterns without the usual error-correction. Thus we might expect fluctuating thresholds to both protect variants from correction and to actually generate more variants.

Though recorded from the scalp, the electroencephalogram is a spatial average of much cortical electrical activity (especially synaptic potentials) in the superficial layers. While reminiscent of stochastic resonance, speeding up darwinian competitions could be done by excitability fluctuations, raising the question of whether some EEG component reflects the equivalent of a forcing function, analogous to climate change.

ONE MIGHT REASONABLY SUPPOSE that a *bottleneck* is my gateway in the hexagonal barrier, and that an *empty niche* is all that unrecruited territory that lies beyond, available for organization via creeping triangular arrays. A reasonable assumption, but nonetheless wrong. They are population-level terms in evolutionary biology, invented long ago and with well-established connotations, that may prove relevant to the dynamics of partitioning neocortex for hexagonal patterns.

A bottleneck refers to small populations that were once large and diverse. Small populations have much less genetic diversity and inbreeding diminishes it further. Should this population somehow expand to a much larger population, as happened with the immigrants across the Bering Straits about 15,000 years ago who eventually colonized all of North and South America, its gene pool will also lack the diversity of the large original population. This is the founder effect — though the expansion itself may preserve any new recombination variants that happen via the boomtime survivals that would otherwise have been lost to juvenile mortality).

A population of clones lacks the variations of most natural populations, what causes us to talk of gene frequencies. But an active hexagonal mosaic need not be uniform. Think of the

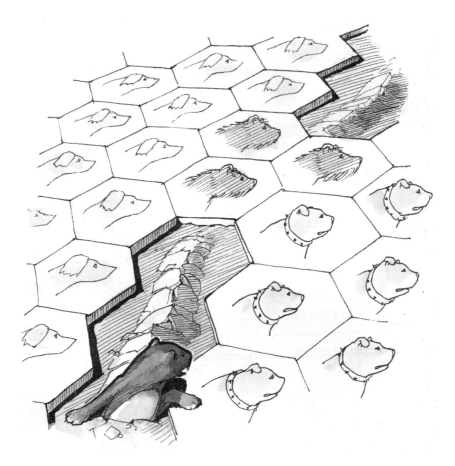

barriers to annexation (and error correction) not as fences or curbs but as little ridge lines — in the park reverie, they might be created by that enterprising gopher burrowing along under the flat surface, so invitingly prepared for pavers. Even if they are flattened down again, they seem to pop up elsewhere. This makes possible an occasional gateway (a flat-enough area between ridgelines). And that produces an occasional variant by preventing error correction from operating. At any one point in time, the cerebral park's paver population exhibits variation. You'd even expect its temporary alcoves to develop regional sub-species, just as a natural population of fruit flies in Hawaii tends to have somewhat different gene pools in different valleys.

So, too, excitability declines in some regions of cortex will wipe out the local triangular array nodes and prevent new ones from forming — in effect, raising a barrier to further cloning. As long as this bumpy landscape keeps changing faster than the most efficient error correction can conform the entire population, there will always be some variation around. If error correction were to triumph everywhere, it would constitute a bottleneck as severe as that of the single pregnant female that finds an empty island, even if the cloned territory is large. Yes, variation will return shortly after some new barriers arise, but its base will be the standardized spatiotemporal pattern rather than that of the more diverse assemblage that preceded the bottlenecking uniformity.

Even a uniform bottleneck hexagonal mosaic (say, *Beethoven* clones occupying hundreds of hexagons) can create variation as it tries to embed a new attractor in the underlying connectivities. Because hexagonal territories have stopped expanding at many different places in the past, the underlying connectivities vary over a mosaic's current territory. To the extent that the old embedded attractors interact with the new one, regional variants will occur *later*, when the Beethoven spatiotemporal pattern is recreated from scratch.

SIMILARLY, AN EMPTY NICHE is not just an unorganized region of cortex. Even busy areas could also have an empty niche — which brings us back once again to multifunctionality.

Niche is an ecological term that refers to all of the resources, protection from predators, nesting sites, and other things that allow a population to reproduce itself; toads might not need waterholes all the time, but a return to the water's edge is essential at egg-laying time and that makes waterholes a part-time but essential element of their niche. A niche is the "outward projection of the needs of an organism."

An empty niche is a term referring to a niche with significant resources that are going unused; lots may be going on in a cortical region but an additional hexagonal resonance is available that, if activated, would cause minimal impact on the other ongoing activities. Mayr describes one extracranial empty niche:

The tropical forests of Borneo and Sumatra, for instance, provide resources for 28 species of woodpeckers. By contrast there are no woodpeckers what-so-ever in the exceedingly similar forests of New Guinea, and on that island hardly any other species of birds make use of the woodpecker niche. The existence of insufficiently utilized resources is further documented by successful cases of colonization or invasion which do not result in a visible decline of any previously existing species.

Most species are relatively independent of one another, simply getting out of one another's way like the proverbial two ships passing in the night — but without even the distant wave of a hand.

So too, we might find that the different species of cortical spatiotemporal melodies can, if point-to-area inhibition is also low, occupy the same cortex without significant interaction: perhaps those competing *Bach* and *Beethoven* hexagons can overlap just as French and Dutch do in Belgium. Avoiding using the same minicolumns would presumably aid "bilingualism"; changing the slant of the triangular arrays, earlier discussed for the passive resonances (p. 73), may also be a possible method for active spatiotemporal patterns to avoid one another.

As Mayr points out elsewhere, the "existence of such potential niche space explains, of course, why speciation is sometimes successful." To make an economic analogy, we might say that there was an *unfilled* niche for spreadsheet software prior to 1980 and that the boom in spreadsheets was a speciation event as well as an invention. But the *empty* niche concept, per se, is more closely associated with deme extinctions (a regional subpopulation dies out, usually from climate change or infectious disease) where proven-in-the-past resources are now going unused. Subsequent pioneers to this territory may thereby enjoy a boom time.

Some analogies to economics and politics may make this clearer. A classical hidden agenda is encouraging bankruptcies by predatory pricing; it's a stage-setting strategy for a market takeover that establishes a monopoly. The political equivalent might be unrealistic promises of tax cuts, or denigrating all government accomplishments ("Can't do anything right").

Although it seems paradoxical to hear aspiring politicians say this, the governing niche itself won't be destroyed by this anarchistic maneuver. That's because our society has become too complex to run without government services and, in a fast-moving world, the government pays for the long-term research that no corporation has the incentive to perform itself. But even a smaller pie may be very profitable for the supporters of such anarchist politicians, particularly when the benefits are largely disguised, usually by shifting the tax burden to others. (As the lawyers like to say, *Cui bono*? The more pointed journalistic version of "Who benefits?" is "Follow the money.") One has to imagine such contractions of business or government as being temporary, likely followed by a re-expansion around a new base, refilling the niche — and ask what that base of expansion will center about (likely — though not inevitably — the well-situated survivors). So too, in this neocortical theory, we see the possibilities for establishing sizeable pluralities, both by direct competition and by better surviving environmental fluctuations.

Here, even when a pattern falls temporarily silent, the ghostly blackboard of temporarily enhanced connectivity makes it possible for the pattern to again ignite. And perhaps booting up with a novel pattern, a composite of several patterns that had recently inhabited the territory — but never simultaneously. Although I doubt that it is the most elementary mechanism for category formation, overlain hexagons hold the promise of dealing with advanced levels of abstraction.

What makes the wasp's behavior more like that of a computer than an architect is the lack of any comprehension of the goal. Instead, the insect focuses on a series of immediate tasks. This distinction between "local" tasks, which could be accomplished by innate programming alone, and "global" goals, which may require a more complete perspective and understanding of the need a behavior serves, will be crucial to our analyses of more complex behavior.

JAMES L. GOULD and CAROL GRANT GOULD, 1994

Instead of thoughts of concrete things patiently following one another in a beaten track of habitual suggestion, we have the most abrupt cross-cuts and transitions from one idea to another, the most rarefied abstractions and discriminations, the most unheard-of combinations of elements, the subtlest associations of analogy; in a word, we seem suddenly introduced into a seething caldron of ideas, where everything is fizzling and bobbing about in a state of bewildering activity, where partnerships can be joined or loosened in an instant, treadmill routine is unknown, and the unexpected seems the only law. According to the idiosyncrasy of the individual, the scintillations will have one character or another. They will be sallies of wit and humor; they will be flashes of poetry and eloquence; they will be constructions of dramatic fiction or of mechanical devices, logical or philosophic abstractions, business projects, or scientific hypotheses, with trains of experimental consequences based thereon; they will be musical sounds, or images of plastic beauty or picturesqueness, or visions of moral harmony. But, whatever their differences may be, they will all agree in this – that their genesis is sudden and, as it were, spontaneous.

WILLIAM JAMES, 1880

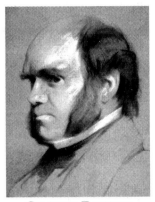

CHARLES DARWIN

T HIS IS THE FIRST JUNCTURE at which we can see all six essentials of a darwinian process (p. 21) emerge from the hexagonal cloning theory for a neocortical patchwork quilt. So indulge me in a little celebratory recapitulation about principles before we delve more deeply into their products. The six essentials are:

1. *There is a characteristic pattern involved.* We have identified a pattern (spatiotemporal firing pattern within a "0.5 mm" hexagon in the superficial layers of neocortex) that can be standardized in a crystalline manner. The pattern is as abstract as a bar code; just as the DNA string looks nothing like a folded protein, these cerebral codes bear little resemblance to the objects or movements they represent.

2. *The pattern must be copied somehow (indeed, that which is copied may serve to define the pattern).* Copying identified a

way of compacting the essential Hebbian cell-assembly, and its connectivity changes, into only two adjacent 0.5 mm hexagons of neocortex. Thanks to the point-to-annulus tendencies of the same neurons that recurrently excite one another, two adjacent "parent" neurons seem capable of entraining a third and fourth to initiate a triangular array, one that can be extended for some distance. But the overall effect is to clone the spatiotemporal pattern of all the active triangular arrays within a hexagonal-shaped area; thus we can often speak of hexagonal cloning. Even noncloning hexagons may have an important function: to serve as a barrier.

3. *Variant patterns must sometimes be produced by chance.* Variants can be generated by relaxing error correction at gateways through the barriers. But superpositions readily occur; because these patterns are a fairly sparse fill of the hexagon, the superpositions may be able to code for supersets such as categories, sensory-motor associations, and even relations between relations such as syntax and metaphor. It all doesn't have to be crammed into one hexagon because "message digest" hashes may suffice to call forth the "full text" from elsewhere.

4. *The pattern and its variants must compete with one another for occupation of a limited work space.* Indeed, with end runs around barriers, competition is hard to avoid. The cortex is certainly limited, just as is a patchwork quilt. The work space is probably the equivalent of that paved park, with its alcoves in which demes can go extinct. Whether all neocortex functions this way or whether specialization may often prevent cloning competitions is an empirical question to be answered as experimental resolution improves.

5. *The competition is biased by a multifaceted environment, for example, how often the grass is watered, cut, fertilized, and frozen, giving one pattern more of the work space than another.* No, we haven't yet identified which cortical pattern is the crabgrass. But long-term memory is a memorized environment (via connectivity changes that create basins

of attraction). Sensory inputs from our real-time physical environment (and more distant cortical inputs) should be able to bias resonances without actually cloning distinctive spatiotemporal patterns. Short-term memories in the form of fading basins of attraction, established by cloned patterns a few minutes earlier, can form part of this environment and so facilitate stage-setting moves.

6. *There is a skewed survival to reproductive maturity (environmental selection is mostly juvenile mortality) or a skewed distribution of those adults who successfully mate (sexual selection), so new variants always preferentially occur around the more successful of the current patterns.* Nothing I've said so far has demonstrated that the more populous patterns have a tendency to generate most of the next generation's variants — but perhaps you've guessed why. It's the ubiquitous surface-to-volume ratio relationship that provides Darwin's inheritance principle. In a basically two-dimensional world such as retina or cortex, it's called the perimeter-to-area relationship. Bigger areas have more edge, and the edges are where error correction can be escaped more easily, thanks to the very excitability fluctuations that help make the margins marginal. So the more successful patterns tend to be the base from which most variants form.

So far, so good. But what about those five additional features that influence the rate of evolutionary change? Happily, we can also see stability plus the four "catalysts" that speed evolution in this same neocortical patchwork quilt:

7. *Stability may occur, as in getting stuck in a rut (a local minima in the adaptational landscape). Variants occur but they backslide easily.* An even background of excitation that avoids the formation of barriers seems a good setup for achieving a stable uniform wallpaperlike pattern. More in a minute.

8. *Systematic recombination generates many more variants than do copying errors and the far-rarer point mutations.* An end run around a barrier demonstrates one way for variants to met

up with clones of their parents. Recombination can occur at those frontiers where different spatiotemporal patterns meet. Though the no-mans-land hexagons, surrounded as they are, are unlikely to start cloning unoccupied territory, the back-and-forth of the frontier leaves behind a composite attractor that could subsequently be activated if the parent active patterns died out in the region.

9. *Fluctuating environments (seasons, climate changes, diseases) change the name of the game, shaping up more complex patterns capable of doing well in several environments. For such jack-of-all-trades selection to occur, the climate must change much faster than efficiency adaptations can track it.* Fluctuating excitability is highly likely, just from the EEG evidence, and, because its time scale is the milliseconds of the PSPs, it is indeed much faster than the minutes-long LTP mechanisms of neocortex that alter the basins of attraction, sometimes permanently. Thus in cortex, we have the essential setup for evolving elaborate patterns offline, ones that are well in excess of current behavioral requirements.

10. *Parcellation, as when rising sea level converts the hilltops of one large island into an archipelago of small islands, typically speeds evolution.* As threshold levels rise or background excitation fades, there are many opportunities for chopping up neocortical territories with noncloning barriers.

11. *Local extinctions (as when an island population becomes too small to sustain itself) speed evolution because they create empty niches.* In the systematic recombination explanation above, there were ghostly patterns in the connectivity, lingering after the active spatiotemporal patterns had been died out. Should an active pattern come close to this basin of attraction and start up its spatiotemporal pattern in two adjacent hexagons, it could clone away without any competition for awhile. For a novel pattern, that could represent the chance to "establish itself" — and some variants.

There are also catalysts acting at several removes, just as in Darwin's example of how cats could improve the clover, and we have no difficulty imagining how this could happen with cortical work spaces. Cloning competitions at the object level could occasionally overrun another competition at the event or metaphor level.

IT IS USEFUL TO LOOK FOR BIOLOGICAL ANALOGIES, for some of the reasons that I noted at the beginning of the last chapter, but one shouldn't expect to find perfect parallels. For example, the cortex may well be the appropriate home for Lamarckism (the pre-darwinian notion that skills acquired during life can be somehow fed back to the genes, and so inherited by one's offspring). In cortex, after all, there are generations of lateral copying attempts, and their improved versions can feed back into the connectivity changes to influence what happens tomorrow when another copying attempt is made. In biology, what's wrong with Lamarckism is the Weismannian genotype-phenotype barrier, the difficulty of making chimeras, and a distinct individual that survives as a cohesive unit. So far, the cortex only has a copying unit (the hexagonal activity doesn't always live and die as a unit, though embedded attractors encourage that) and it readily produces chimeras with hybrid vigor in a most unbiological way.

You can, of course, ask: Does capture by an attractor constitute stabilizing selection? Does the hexagon correspond to an allele of a gene? A genome (one average organism's worth of genes)? Even a population can potentially be a unit of selection in biology. But here, much as I like finding traditional parallels, I suspect that we are better off focusing instead on the neural substrate — such as the geometry, chaos, and connectivity concepts of the last few chapters — rather than seriously seeking parallels in other levels of biology. We have profited from importing island biogeography concepts, even if our hot-spot islands also grow via dendritic amplification mechanisms and raise their sea levels via AGCs. So, too, we may profit from asking about clades, neutral evolution, evolutionarily stable strategies, and (coming up in chapter 8) sexual selection.

But we shouldn't expect an exact mapping of either the immune system or cortical darwinian dynamics onto the individuals-that-copy-and-die framework that biological evolution has settled into. Yes, they all feature the darwinian process — yet the darwinian process isn't really an analogy: it's a crank for complexity that can be turned by instability, whenever a mechanism exists that implements all six essentials. This process just happens to be a major law of the universe, right up there with chemical bonds as a prime generator of interesting combinations, and one apparently able to run on different substrates, each with their own distinctive properties that may, or may not, correspond to those seen elsewhere.

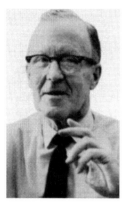

HEBB'S DISCOVERY OF THE CELL-ASSEMBLY is not only a useful historical tidbit for the intermission, but his concerns about what he perceived as failures of his cell-assembly theory may help us judge the strengths and weaknesses of my competing hexagons.

What got Hebb to thinking about cell-assemblies was the problem of perception and thought. When, in 1938, Lorente de Nó suggested how cerebral cortex could generate sustained activity with reverberating circuits, he opened up some new possibilities, ones that had seemed closed since Sherrington's day. Hebb wanted a way to think about reactivating a memory trace by thought, without a new sensory stimulus interceding. Lorente's idea gave him sustained activity (the first reason he needed chains of many neurons), but Hebb was still worried about how objects seen from different perspectives were nonetheless perceived as the same object. He considered it a failing of his 1945–1949 cell-assembly theory that it couldn't handle such a key property of concepts.

DONALD O. HEBB

Experimental work in Hebb's own lab in Montreal about 1960 eventually provided evidence for various specialized groups participating in what seemed to be a unitary percept, such as that of a triangle or square. It was a surprise finding from quite a different experiment. The physiological tremor of the eyeball is called micronystagmus; it causes a light-dark boundary in the image to sweep back and forth over a band as wide as a half-dozen photoreceptors. That can potentially smear the image quite a bit. You can, however, force the image to move with the eye by

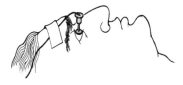

an ingenious system of mounting the square or triangle just in front of a contact lens. Whenever the eye moves, so does its target — and so the image is stabilized on the retina.

But what happened was not that the image became sharper. Instead, the subject reported that the image was incomplete; parts of it had a mysterious tendency to fade away and then reappear. In a series of six presentations, controlled by turning on a little light bulb that was also getting a free ride from the eye's movements, the triangle might lose one or another of its three sides. Squares had similar problems, and even faded out entirely on some of the presentations. Images of a face would sometimes lose a nose or eye. I seem to remember, in the excitement over this in the early 1960s (one of the reasons that I switched about then from physics into neurophysiology), that someone claimed to have finally seen a Cheshire Cat doing its disappearing act.

Hubel and Wiesel's orientation-sensitive cortical neurons, found about the same time, suggested an obvious mechanism. Together with the Cheshire Cat fade outs, they resolved the theoretical failing that Hebb identified. It also gave him another reason

[This time the cat] vanished quite slowly, beginning with the end of the tail, and ending with the grin, which remained some time after the rest of it had gone.

"Well! I've often seen a cat without a grin," thought Alice; "but a grin without a cat! It's the most curious thing I ever saw in my life!"

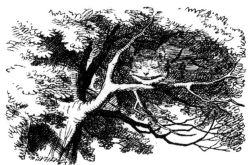

why a cell-assembly of multiple cortical neurons would be needed: to handle all the line orientations that form the outline of an object.

In retrospect, this committee of feature detectors was the most important reason for a cell-assembly. Lorente's reverberating circuits may have gotten Hebb to thinking about neuronal ensembles about 1940, but they really aren't needed to get sustained activity — something we only learned about in the early 1960s, once we were able to control the firing rate of a single neuron during intracellular recording.

All of Hebb's arguments and evidence (summarized in his 1980 book, *Essay on Mind*) carry over to my more restricted notion of a hexagonal cell-assembly. My triangular arrays add quite a bit of redundancy but their interdigitation also serves to "compress the code" into a half-mm hexagonal space. Such concentrating of the elements allows for lots of little local neural circuits to form, and perhaps change some synaptic strengths in a long-lasting manner. Hebb's dual trace memory is thereby implemented: any adjacent pair of these hexagonal circuits could later reconstitute the firing pattern in all of the multiple triangular arrays that were originally formed during the original stimulus presentation.

Hebb unfortunately died in 1985, well before I figured this out. He might have liked how his dual memory traces, his synapses strengthened by success, and his cell-assemblies all came to theoretically hang together in a little hexagon.

JUST AS THE FIRST ACT introduces the cast and poses the problems, so the second act tends to show the surprising consequences. My second act is about the possible products of a fast-acting darwinian principle in neocortex, things such as categories, metaphors, good guesses, and the train of thought. I'll start with Hebb's triangle generalization problem and some static-seeming super-positions of schemas, but it's all dynamic underneath: keep James's train of thought in mind, that series of mental states that preceded your current one, each one fading into the background but overlain on its predecessors — and all capable of contributing to what connections you're likely to make right now.

Just imagine those various fading attractors as like that Japanese technique of finely slicing some raw fish, then tilting the block sideways (fallen dominos are another analogy, if you are sashimi impaired). The bottom layer may be hardest to reach but it goes back furthest. Stage-setting with multiple layers of fading schemas may be handy for promoting creativity, getting the right layers of attractors in about the right order and so adjusting their relative strengths. (I can hear it now: *The Sashimi Theory of Creativity*, a suitably raw successor to all those half-baked right-brain schemes).

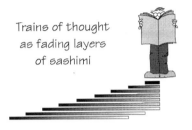

Trains of thought as fading layers of sashimi

But such histories can also be distracting, and we often try to let them fade, try to avoid reexciting them with further thinking. There are various mind-clearing techniques (I take half-hour naps, myself). My friend Don Michael suggests that forming large quasi-stable hexagonal territories might be what meditation with a mantra is all about, preempting the everyday concerns that would otherwise partition the work space and plate out new short-term attractors. By replacing it all with the mantra's nonsense pattern, and holding it long enough for neocortical LTP to fade, the meditator gets a fresh start (for things other than the mantra!). Sounds good to me, but you might forget your grocery list if you carry it too far.

An ordinary mantra won't, of course, wipe the work space clean: to prematurely erase those fading attractors, you'll need a fancier mantra that disrupts instead. Short of fogging with seizures, as in electroshock therapy, I don't know of any such eraser schemas — though one can imagine mental viruses that might preempt entry into those fading basins of attraction, more analogous to an obscuring coat of paint than to a true eraser.

A NEUROPHYSIOLOGICAL THEORY of higher intellectual function is the focus of the rest of this book. Ultimately, it's about consciousness (as the currently dominant patch of the quilt!). Though you'll never encounter such a list in most of the popular and academic books about consciousness, any such theory is going to need to account for:

How items of our vocabularies are represented.

How memories are stored and recalled.

How darwinian shaping-up takes place.

How "new ideas" arise, perhaps as pattern variants.

Those four, at least, have pretty much fallen out of our search for the darwinian essentials. The rest are harder:

The existence of hallucinations and dreams.

Déjà vu experiences. Abnormally widespread cloning of an input pattern (perhaps due to lack of competition) might produce the conscious experience usually associated with strong memory resonances that allow widespread cloning. *Jamais vu* unfamiliarity with the familiar would also be nice to explain.

Unreliable memories. Because the long-term synaptic connectivities can be modified by a new active pattern, this could often happen; to avoid this rewriting of history, the subcortical regulation of the cortical competitions probably includes giving permission for the modification of connectivities. Similarly, we'd like something appropriate for concrete thinking and the *idée fixe.*

How abstractions and categories are represented and created. In particular, a theory of mind needs structures suitable for schemas, scripts, syntax, and metaphors.

How the various connotations of a word such as "comb" are linked, given that they're likely stored in different cortical areas.

The presence of specialized cortical regions that can also participate in nonspecialist tasks.

The ability to hold a behavioral set, after selecting it from among possibilities. What might an agenda look like?

Subconscious shaping up, while one's attention seems directed elsewhere.

Creation of efficient subroutines that function outside of conscious processing, something suitable for Zen archery. A "well-grooved" pattern might "play" from a small cortical territory, like the roll for a player piano, to tie a necktie without competing in the playoffs for consciousness. We do, after all, occasionally manage to do two things at the same time.

Serial-order specialties for language and speculative planning, not to mention all the small muscle sequencing that a child needs to tie a shoelace.

Speed-of-thought correlates, mechanisms that could vary from time to time in the same individual. During the transitions of manic-depressive illness, a person can go from a fluidity of making connections and decisions to a slow, labored train of thought that lingers too long and fails to make obvious connections. And back again.

Our passion for discovering patterns. In our first year of life, we discovered phonemes within words. A year later, we were busy discovering schemas and syntax within sentences, and then we went on to discover narrative principles among more extended discourses.

The impression of a narrator, juggling decisions, and speculating about tomorrow. Any explanation needs to be consistent with the neurological evidence that no partial cortical lesion abolishes the "self."

That's the kind of coverage needed for a useful theory of mind. It may not have to explain all of two centuries of neurology, one century of psychology, and a half-century of neurobiology and cognitive neuroscience — but it can't be truly inconsistent with *any* of it. A theory of mind needs a lot of explanatory power, while still being specific enough to make experimental predictions.

THEORETICAL EDIFICES have held some surprises in evolutionary theory, quite aside from all the emergent phenomena. For example, one is accustomed to thinking that, if a piece of the foundation fails, the whole edifice collapses and should be abandoned. But that isn't necessarily true when dealing with robust processes such as Darwin's; one can be wrong about elements of the foundation (as Darwin himself was about inheritance in 1859, as Clerk Maxwell was in 1865 about the ether) and still gain many insights about superstructure.

Darwin didn't know about Mendel's genes; he thought in terms of blending inheritance, not the particulate inheritance that went on to find its basis in DNA segments called alleles. Although I will use triangular arrays from recurrent excitation and their resulting hexagons as my examples in the coming chapters about the cognitive implications of darwinism in the brain, remember that other mechanisms might prove to be the foundation of what is copied with inherited variation in our neocortex. I'm trying to piece together a general theory for how the superficial layers of neocortex could run the darwinian ratchet, but I'm also — in *Act II* — carrying on William James's project, attempting to show how any such darwinian theory could account for higher intellectual function.

As I give examples of how categories could be created, and elaborated into schemas and metaphors, try to distinguish the emergent structures per se — and perhaps guess how they could be implemented with different darwinian building materials, ones that still satisfy the six essentials and provide a few accelerating factors in the manner of my triangular arrays and hexagonal mosaics.

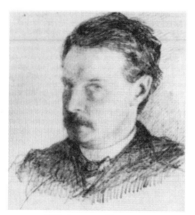

WILLIAM JAMES
(self portrait, 1873)

Act II

I suggest that memory is organized with a framework of motor programs within the brain. Far from being a black box of no relevance to behaviorist psychology, the brain is a jack-in-the-box, filled to the brim with spring-loaded plans of action. As such it is the very wellspring of all behavior. These brain-mind behavior programs, like sensory representations, are virtual — and they have even been called "fictive" to capture their promissory aspect — but they are no less real. In our being and becoming, they are us and we are they.

J. ALLAN HOBSON, 1994

Rejection [of the idea that mental events have no locus] by common sense, for whatever reason, proves nothing. Other fields of science are built on propositions that may seem absurd but in fact are true. (Air is heavy, has weight? Water is made up of two gases? The continents are adrift in the oceans?)

DONALD O. HEBB, 1980

7

The Brownian Notion

No image could ever be adequate to the concept of a
triangle in general. It would never attain that
universality of the concept which renders it valid of all
triangles, whether right-angled, obtuse-angled, or
acute-angled; it would always be limited to a part only
of this sphere. The schema of the triangle can exist
nowhere but in thought.

IMMANUEL KANT, 1781

STARTING THE SECOND ACT WITH KANT'S TRIANGLES is my way
of reminding myself of the importance of how you pose the
questions — and how "answers" often reformulate a
question rather than answering it. We reposition the foundations
beneath our feet as we grope for a firmer footing. This is
particularly evident when we deal with abstractions, when we
move beyond the representations of our sensory worlds and of
our movements and operate in the realm of meta-representations,
such as categories or analogies.

But there are some problems with this. When I was first
exposed to the problem of generalizing about specific examples of
triangles, I was fresh from a course in set theory, and so "spring
loaded" to find subsets and supersets as I looked for a mechanistic
foundation for such mental categories (as you'll see, I might have
been better off taking a music appreciation course instead).
Things look very different to me today, in large part because of
developments in cognitive science involving categorical perception, grammar, schemas, scripts, and metaphors. Darwinian

copying competitions, in turn, have provided me with another place to stand, a different footing from which to view all of those various types of categories — and an ability to imagine how we might construct them "on the fly," even invent new levels of abstraction.

THE NATURE OF CATEGORIES has been discussed at least since the ancient Greeks, but the darwinian process provides a fresh way of looking at them.

Yes, the category is a class but there's often a prototype — a primitive example that shares a lot of features with other members. Eleanor Rosch talks of a basic level category, such as "dog," that's defined by the ease with which children and new-comers acquire the concept. Above this is a superordinate level with more abstract classes, such as "mammal" and "pet." Below the basic level is a subordinate level, subclasses such as "German Shepherd."

Unique individuals, to which we give proper names such as "Fido," may be difficult class-of-one categories, requiring much more information, such as the features that distinguish that individual from all others of the class. One should not assume — as I did, fresh from set theory — that individuals or episodes are the primitive unit memories, out of which classes are built. With some exceptions such as an infant's representation of his mother, the unique individual is probably a late stage of category construction, subject to more errors than the populous categories. A

> A thing "is" whatever it gives us least trouble to think it is. There is no other "is" than this.
>
> SAMUEL BUTLER (II)

unit memory is often more like a forest than an individual tree — and that means there is no firm line between representations and meta-representations.

Most unit memories are probably the fuzzier categories and their associations, not our societal and set theory units. As Bickerton observes, "Without categories, there can be nothing to attach symbols to, since linguistic symbols, as has been apparent at least since Saussure, do not relate directly to objects in the world, but rather to our concepts of the generalized classes to which raw objects belong. Without associations between stimuli (rather than merely between stimulus and response), there would be no way in which symbols could be attached reliably to concepts." To use words in a referential manner, you've got to recognize them as more than mere labels for objects. They have to be treated as abstract units in a hierarchial network of meanings. And meaning, to the followers of Jean Piaget, is inseparable from experience — meanings are constructed.

ASSOCIATIONS BETWEEN UNIT MEMORIES are, moreover, a test of representation schemes, such as my spatiotemporal firing pattern within a neocortical hexagon, as associations, too, must produce representations under some conditions. An association between various representations, as in the various connotations of a word such as "comb," might be expressed as physical contiguity or overlap:

- o   a *cluster* of representations, in the manner of photographs grouped together on a bulletin board,
- o   a *concatenation* of representations, in the manner of genes strung together on a chromosome, or
- o   a *composite* made by superposition of representations, in the manner of a double exposure, pastiche, or chimera.

But physical contiguity might not be needed. To what extent might a virtual construction suffice? Mere linkages, as in a distributed data base, parts of which are maintained in diverse locations and assembled only when needed? What would bind them together, in the manner of those colored strings on school bulletin boards that lead to the portraits of the members of the committee?

I suspect that the categories we often use, like those that birds and monkeys can learn, are simpler than the ones that fill the remaining chapters. Feature detection is often fuzzy, with a wide range of acceptable shapes still yielding the same perception — which is, of course, serving the function of categorization. But some of these crude mechanisms may not be very extensible, as they say in the software business. Simple foundations may suffice for limited purposes but other foundations may prove better when

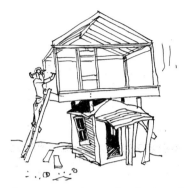

you go to add on a second story (in archaeology, a ruin's wall thickness is considered a clue to its original height).

Relationships, too, are abstractions, ones that particularly concern perspective and orientation, or how we frame and punctuate messages. Analogies, metaphors, similes, parables, and mental models involve the *comparing* of relationships, as when we make an imperfect analogy between *is-bigger-than* and *is-faster-than*, by inferring that *bigger-is-faster*.

Given that we seem capable of endless levels of abstraction and haven't yet run out of coding space, we may require a representation scheme that is dimensionally similar for both the elementary (apple) and the high-order (Impressionist Still Life). Happily, in *gedankenexperiments*, hexagons for cerebral codes seem capable (to anticipate chapter 10) of handling any level of abstraction, meta-metaphors and beyond — even representing the *gedankenexperiment* itself.

Let us begin with a new category arising from a darwinian competition, order emerging from disorder — what my friend Doug vanderHoof promptly labeled "the Brownian notion" on the analogy to the random movement of dust particles in a beam of sunlight — and the way they can eventually coalesce into "dust bunnies" that lurk in undisturbed corners.

ASSOCIATIVE MEMORY IS A BIG SUBJECT and I don't propose to explain why Pavlov's dog learned to associate the dinner bell with the subsequent appearance of food (there are, one suspects, lots of subcortical ways of doing that). Fancy explanations (such as hexagonal mosaic competitions) aren't needed for associations per se: very simple invertebrates do associations, even within a single second-order neuron. Nor are fancy explanations needed for categories, as such.

Cerebral cortex, however, has the reputation for doing particularly intricate associative memory tasks, especially in the neocortex that mammals have developed so highly. The superficial layers of neocortex certainly look, from *Act I*, as if they could run a full-fledged darwinian process at the population level, mimicking the more familiar darwinian processes that operate on longer time scales. This goes far beyond, and seems more robust, than anything that I can imagine emerging from a revisionist two-maps loop. That my neocortical Darwin Machine doesn't maintain a germ line, but instead looks Larmarkian enough to overlay even inborn wiring patterns, is a very desirable feature for the seat of cultural evolution. Presumably some cortical areas are less plastic than others, retaining most of their innate attractors over the years.

The cloning competition probably isn't needed as an immediate prelude for making a decision, not for most perceptual tasks or movement programs. The tasks illustrated so far, movement choice and ambiguous object recognition, are well within the capabilities of all of our primate cousins, even tree shrews. The question is whether a Darwin Machine might facilitate higher intellectual function: our syntactic language, our abilities to plan grocery lists and careers, our fondness for making music, for inventing new games to play, and for automatically detecting new patterns among established relationships.

Patterns within patterns is what syntax is all about, what the two-year-old child is detecting via listening before bursting into full sentences with appropriate syntax (and with relatively little overt trial and error). Relations among relations are what metaphor is all about. They're far more abstract than anything that our closest cousins seem to do, though skillful teachers of apes may yet demonstrate that the ape brain is capable of handling the task. Apes could, for example, merely lack the child's acquisitiveness for words and their interrelations. Absence of evidence, as the archaeologists are fond of noting, is not evidence of absence.

SUPERPOSITIONS ARE CAPABLE OF DOING ASSOCIATIONS within my hexagons framework, and we have already seen how one spatio-temporal pattern may overlay another at a frontier between two competing patterns. There is a row of hexagons getting both patterns in various ratios; I usually slip into talking of them "competing" for the space, but they might simply overlap (their triangular arrays might interdigitate without interaction, just as in my example of compacting a Hebbian cell-assembly on p. 46).

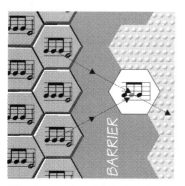

The main problem is whether such overlapped hexagons could ever have an independent existence, that is, be able to clone their own territory and compete. This borderline row is, after all, flanked by already established patterns, limiting its reproductive possibilities in a manner reminiscent of hybrid sterility. Let me illustrate two ways to enlarge this thin belt of composite hexagons and improve the hybrid's chances for having viable offspring.

A barrier needs to be thicker if the axons have more than one cluster of terminals on integer repeats (as some clearly do). Thin regions of barrier can then become gateways.

Intrinsic horizontal axons are often longer than 0.5 mm, with additional terminals clustering around integer multiples of the local metric. Error correction comes not only from the six immediate neighbors but potentially from another six backing them up. This means that barriers may need to be thicker if error correction is to be escaped.

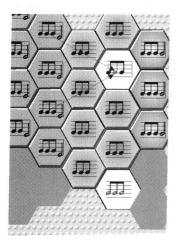

But it also means that the no-mans-land of composites may be a few units wide, enough for a little territory of its own if it resonated sufficiently, perhaps one that could survive better than either of the originals. If barriers were appropriately located, one can imagine the hybrid colonizing new territory by spreading out the narrow end of the composite territory.

Frontiers sweeping back-and-forth are the other setup for wide belts of composite hexagons, provided they have lingering effects. Think of Alsace, where both French and German are spoken, thanks to the fluctuations of the French-German frontier (four times in the last century). Or, as mentioned earlier, those parts of Belgium speaking both French and Dutch. Louvain — or, if you prefer, Leuven — is said to "be on the language border" but both languages are mutually understood over a much wider belt. The back-and-forth of hexagonal frontiers could leave a "multilingual" belt that is much wider than the no-mans-land of today's competition.

Note that the first type of belt is in the manner of jam sessions in jazz, operating directly at the level of active cloning of spatiotemporal patterns, overlaying one melody on another. You might acquire a new movement program that allowed you to pat your head and rub your stomach at the same time. But my second wider-belt scheme relies on an intermediary, that of forming a new attractor in the connectivity itself. This could happen without the two active patterns ever being present at the same time (indeed, even if the programs were ordinarily competitors). The novelty starts at the level of attractors, rather than that of performance, almost as if one sheet of music had been photocopied on top of another, and someone then tried to play the composite.

Most such superpositions are, of course, unplayable — but not all, and darwinian processes are quite capable of discarding the chaff and retaining the workable for further rounds of variation, shaping up higher quality entities. As work spaces turn over, superpositions ought to happen all the time, as ghostly attractors linger after the synchronized triangular arrays have been silenced. This could function much like the exchange of genetic material between species via retroviruses. Just think of how Charles Ives used those musical snippets, conditioning what followed with the fading attractors of *Yankee Doodle*.

Species that are competitors over ecological time may be mutualists over evolutionary time, each providing a store of genetic variation that can be tapped by the other.

ROBERT HOLT, 1990

Basins of attraction, because of their afore-mentioned tendency to capture different initial conditions, have that important feature of a loose-fitting category: the resulting activity pattern is about the same, so the significance is about the same. As Walter Freeman notes:

> [N]eocortex may have one or more global attractors with multiple wings. State transitions may occur as brief confinements to a wing of an attractor, followed by release to another....The concept of an attractor and its attendant basin is too rigid, because neocortical dynamics progresses through time by continual changes in state that adapt the cortices to the changing environment. The change constitutes a trajectory in cortical state space, which never returns exactly to a prior state, but which (on receipt of a stimulus, for example) returns sufficiently close to the prior state that cortical output places a target of the transmission into the same basin of attraction as did the prior output.

Such "chaotic itinerancy" might be like the seasonal progress of a peddler, revisiting towns that have changed somewhat since the last visit. Itinerancy emphasizes the recurrence of similar, rather than identical, states.

This brings us back to my sashimi example, where a train of thought serves to stack up fading attractors. This allows a certain type of stage setting move. To access rarely used memories (say, the name of the street just north of your childhood home), it may help to first recall the houses on the block, the playmates, the local school — best of all, the direction on your left as you looked at sunrise. Then, if this stage setting sufficiently molds the approach landscape, you will finally pop into the right basin of attraction and activate the street name's spatiotemporal pattern, its cerebral code. With some luck, you'll be able to get a big enough chorus singing it, and eventually pronounce the word (in my case, "80th Street").

LINGERING BASINS OF ATTRACTION need not be limited to those produced by the triangular arrays within a hexagonal area. A synaptic modification can, for example, provide a customary "groove" that predicts the path of a familiar moving object. One can exploit the time asymmetry of NMDA potentiation; like lingering mouse trails on a computer screen, the enhancement trails the action and doesn't lead it. But on replay, interesting things happen.

Such synaptic enhancement can, in models of repeated trials, convert some "place cells" into "future place cells"(their best response becomes centered slightly downstream of where the moving object is currently located). In a feedback or efference copy system, this offset could tend to move an arm back on to a customary path if it was somewhat off the path. This scheme doesn't demand basins of attraction or hexagonal copying, yet the synaptic modification might well generate them as side effects. It's an empirical question that awaits answers, but much of the nonhexagonal activity probably modifies actual basins of attraction — and thus changes the chances, making some spatio-temporal patterns easier to clone than others, easier to get started *de novo*. And reigniting a code is the cortical equivalent of spontaneous combustion.

The neocortical projections of the entorhinal area and amygdala probably function without creating hexagonal mosaics. (Edelman bravely calls these areas "cortical appendages," thus risking the charge of "Neocorticocentricism!"— but I agree with him for my present purpose of understanding the basis of quality novelty.) Certainly the four widely broadcast neuromodulators (from subcortical neurons having 10 to 100 times more axon terminals per neuron than most) seem to lack the specificity needed to *generate* hexagonal mosaics, yet they might be very effective at biasing the basins of attraction.

It is only recently that scientists were stunned to discover how much is actually going on inside the brain during sleep. Once scientists had gotten used to their counterintuitive discovery that internal brain functions persist at high levels during sleep, they gave up the idea that the brain itself ever really rests. Then some cells were discovered in the pons whose activity decreased to about half during non-REM sleep and was virtually arrested during REM sleep while the rest of the brain was active at near seizure levels. What did the cells contain? Norepinephrine and serotonin — the amines. . . . When we are awake, these cells fire and secrete amines continuously, which among other things restrains the cholinergic system. The biggest clusters of serotonin cells lie right down the middle of the pons, and the norepinephrine cells lie on either side of them. From these sites, they all project great distances all the way up to the cortex and down to the spinal cord. This reach is much more widespread than that of the acetylcholine system.

J. ALLAN HOBSON, 1994

GIVING EXAMPLES OF A CATEGORY can be challenging. Short of selecting a segregated layer, in the modern manner of CAD program superpositions that allow you to extract the plumbing overlay, how do you decompose one of the hexagonal superpositions?

First of all, while the static diagrams needed for tree-based publication resemble sparsely-filled matrices, ours are not static superpositions in the manner of overprinted characters on a dot-matrix printer. They are spatiotemporal patterns, melodies rather than one crashing chord.

Second, we are not dealing with segregating active patterns here; we want to *evoke* patterns from embedded attractors. The issue is how the system can dwell around one attractor out of the many that a connectivity implements, a task not unlike how you start running rather than walking — which is, after all, another wing of the multilobed attractor called locomotion. The exemplars of a category may, in effect, be attractor lobes that we need to enter.

Third, we have the distributed database possibility, where pointers are middlemen that link scattered elements. This suggests a series of different representations of the same thing, some more useful for recognition than for recall. Recall is always more difficult than recognition, so let me postpone the question about evoking exemplars until we look at the types of possible representations of a category.

WE ARE FAMILIAR with the search that goes from titles to abstracts to full texts, but the nervous system may use other principles in-house. Recollect from chapter 1 how a hashed message digest can be used to find the full text in a database. A hash is like a fingerprint, a unique short-form identifier. Hashing indexes a sparsely-filled high-dimensional space of detailed attributes with stand-ins from a more heavily populated low-dimensional space, the elements of which are highly abstract or even random, compared to what they point to.

One simple application is to create a file name that isn't already in use, and also isn't unnecessarily long, since you want a low-dimensional search space that can be scanned rapidly. A hash of a document can simply use the least significant bits of its checksum, or alternatively, the seconds and minutes fields of file creation time stamps. Just check to make sure it isn't already in use; if so, switch to a different hashing technique and try again. A message digest using more elaborate hashing techniques is exquisitely sensitive to small alterations in the full text, while still remaining fairly short.

Recognition in cognition could simply involve hashing the sensory input with the same algorithm used for memorizing — and then seeing whether this hash matches any of the stored ones. This hash algorithm is, of course, not a truncated checksum but simply, like the abstracting algorithm, the sensory processing abstraction procedures developed by that individual earlier in life, which means that they're unique to the individual, that everyone does it differently.

What's likely to be the most useful short form for recalling categories and specifics? A hash is not an abstract, nor is it a short version of the long text that lacks details. An abstract would be the more useful short form on which to build categories. An abstract or prototype category is just the opposite of a message digest, insensitive to details (a basin of attraction allows for the kind of loose fit that an abstract needs).

SUFFICIENT DETAIL FOR RECALL PER SE is, however, another matter. In chapter 5 (p. 95), I discussed the problem of creating a new basin of attraction amidst all the old ones. Remember that every hexagon of the cortical work space has a somewhat different history, because of where frontiers and barriers were located on various past occasions; the *apple* resonance might not overlap everywhere with that of *banana*. Each hexagon has a different sashimi layering, from its particular ghostly blackboard of short-term attractors and from its particular long-term memories.

If copying is not actively maintaining a spatiotemporal pattern with error correction, attractors may alter it to fit a locally embedded one. A pattern close to one of a hexagon's existing attractors will simply be captured, changed to match the one encouraged by an old attractor, and the original lost. It is only in those hexagons where the new pattern doesn't come close to an existing attractor that it stands a chance of being uniquely embedded in the connectivity.

Larger territories make it more likely that a novel spatio-temporal pattern can escape the straightjacket of old attractors, and thus be successfully memorized, for both the short term and the consolidated long term. Note that this accomplishes the same end as hashing's search for an existing match (though it does not guarantee a novel short form version, as a typical hashing procedure does, only facilitates it by using a large cloned territory to try out many different hexagons).

And why a short form, rather than the real thing? Judging from the difficulties of handling a category-of-one, such as a proper name, the details inherent in a long form are likely to involve a merry chase around a number of hexagons or global attractor lobes in the process of developing details. That suggests a lot of stage setting moves to arrive at the correct ones, perhaps successively plating the territory with a number of different active patterns to shape the sashimi layers into such a form that the correct basin of attraction is entered. (Even a book with a good index seems to require a lot of page flipping before locating a quotable long form.)

One doesn't evoke characteristic activity patterns from silence, of course. It's much more likely to start with random firing patterns that converge onto meaningful ones. Such is what giving exemplars of a category could involve: setting the stage for a detailed category with a series of short forms that warm up the orchestra.

THE FIRST FEW "NOTES" of the spatiotemporal "melody" — as in my discussion of training loops as a spatiotemporal mimic of learning in building up episodic memories (p. 85) — might suffice as a unique "hash" identifier if they are repeatable from one occasion to the next and, as a group, exhibit a lot of variation.

Whatever the short-form prompt for the long-form completion, this serves to illustrate how categories (including sequences such as novel movements and episodic memories) might decompose into detailed parts. The category representation simply needs to link the short forms. Because of the arbitrariness of this composite pattern, the superposition can be repeated yet again for a category of categories (say, *food* that includes *fruit* which includes *apple* and *banana*). And again, with *food* a part of *inanimate objects*.

Note that there is nothing here that requires a consistent hierarchy: *apple* and *fruit* could both be full members of *food* even though *apple* is itself a member of *fruit*. The real world is full of category mistakes and full of shortcuts. I imagine that the brain often uses the equivalent of hypertext links: rather than backing up in a tree hierarchy to go down another major branch, we seem to jump between branches like a squirrel. It's disorderly, but quick — and good enough usually suffices.

IN MY MUSICAL ANALOGY, one node of a triangular array is one note on the piano keyboard. The hexagon contains the whole keyboard (though in no particular order). The spatiotemporal pattern within the hexagon is a melody.

It might be a one-finger melody like the seventh-century Gregorian chants, slowly progressing to nearby notes. Or perhaps several notes in this hexagon fire together, like the tenth-century plainsong of the medieval church, where some voices sang a fifth (a 3:2 ratio of frequencies, seven notes apart) or an octave (2:1, twelve notes apart) higher than the others, though still moving in lockstep.

Now consider our problem of the spatiotemporal pattern for a category. It could be similar to overlaying different melodic lines, where two voices do not move in parallel (in European music, this finally occurred in the thirteenth-century). Counterpoint and more complicated aspects of harmony raise issues of what goes together besides those octaves and fifths. For example, in the major and minor scales (the basis of western music starting with the baroque period), only certain notes (7 of the 12 in an octave) are thought to go well enough together to make chords.

Going well together might, of course, not be a matter of actual overlap in performance. Thanks to Hebb's dual trace memory, there's another possibility. It could be a matter of recalling the spatiotemporal pattern from the spatial-only connectivity: yes, you can temporarily overlay anything, but only certain patterns are likely to stick long enough to be recalled a minute later.

Though I intend music only as a teaching analogy, it reminds us that what goes well together must have a basis in the brain, either innate or acquired. It may be that music will aid us in sorting through the many possible local neural circuits within the hexagons of memory, simply because music does reflect something about mind.

MUCH OF THE WORK OF CORTEX probably isn't even triangular (arrays form up because of the superficial pyramidal neurons, which are only about 39 percent of all neocortical neurons), and therefore not represented in this musical framework of notes, chords, counterpoint, and choirs. I have not attempted to account for much cortical detail in this Darwin Machines theory; in particular, I have not tried to account for the perceptual transformations or learning that most neocortical theorists address.

Mine is not a more abstract theory, so much as it is a mechanistic-level theory about abstractions themselves. It can even handle long-distance multimodality categories such as *comb*.

When the theory was in the course of construction, about 1945, I realized that the facts on which the cell-assembly was based also implied the possibility of what I then called a super-ordinate assembly. When a group of assemblies are repeatedly activated, simultaneously or in sequence, those cortical cells that are regularly active following that primary activity may themselves become organized as a superordinate (second-order) assembly. The activity of this assembly then is representative of that combination of events that individually organized the first-order assemblies. After a baby has developed assembly activities for lines of different slope in the visual field and then is repeatedly exposed to some triangular object — to take the simplest possible example — the combinations of activity of the three assemblies may lead to the formation of a higher-order assembly whose activity is the perception of the triangular object rather than its three sides as such. This might be a second-order assembly if the object is seen always in the same orientation, or a third-order assembly formed in the same way by the repeated excitation of second-order assemblies, fired by seeing the object in different orientations.

DONALD O. HEBB, Essay on Mind, 1980

8

Convergence Zones
with a Hint of Sex

> Symbolic information is interpreted because we refuse
> to accept that any input is meaningless. Shown an
> inkblot, we see bats, witches and dragons. This refusal
> to accept that input is noise lies at the root of
> divination by tarot cards, tea leaves, the livers and
> shoulder blades of animals, or the sticks of the *I Ching*.
> JOHN MAYNARD SMITH, 1993

L ONG-DISTANCE COMMUNICATION within the brain has to bear
the task of matching up information across sensory modalities. I say that because, though there are multisensory
neurons in the cortex, the stroke evidence suggests that the
memory traces for the visual aspects of an object are kept pretty
close to visual cortex, while that for auditory aspects of the same
object are kept on the periphery of auditory cortex.

Yet we associate them pretty well, most of the time. Here's
what I said on the subject in *How Brains Think*:

> The really interesting gray matter is that of the cerebral
> cortex, because that's where most of the novel associations are
> thought to be made — where the sight of a comb, say, is
> matched up to the feel of a comb in your hand. The cerebral
> codes for sight and feel are different, but they become
> associated somehow in the cortex, along with those for
> hearing the sound /kōm/ or hearing the characteristic sounds
> that the tines of a comb make when they're plucked. You can,
> after all, identify a comb in any of these ways. It's
> hypothesized that there are specialized places in the cortex,

called "convergence zones for associative memories," where those different modalities come together.

On the production side, you have linked cerebral codes for pronouncing /kōm/ and for generating the movements that manipulate a comb through the hair on your head. So between the sensory version of the word "comb" and the various movement manifestations, we expect to find a dozen different cortical codes associated with combs.

So how do we integrate those separately-stored codes into a master code for *comb*? Or its equivalent, a process somehow able to associate all those aspects with one another?

DISTANCES IN THE BRAIN are enormous, compared to the scale of millimeter-long dendrites. My longest uninterrupted axon is probably the one that runs as a thinner-than-hair thread from the tip of my big toe to the dorsal column nuclei at the top of my neck, the better part of 2,000 mm. Most of the business of deciding to send an impulse off on that long trip is done within a 0.1 mm segment at the beginning of the axon.

It also takes a while to make the trip, and measuring distance in terms of travel time often makes more sense than thinking in terms of miles or kilometers. There are similar considerations in the brain: I suggested earlier (p. 36) that my triangular arrays might be better measured in travel time than in actual distance. Axon conduction velocities vary enormously, even in different branches of the axon of one neuron.

Sending an impulse from one hemisphere to another takes as long as sending it to the spinal cord, even though there is a tenfold difference in distance. That's because the corpus callosum path is so slow. Faster conduction would require more myelin wrapping, so fewer axons would fit in the limited space of the corpus callosum. In the monkey, about 70 percent of the axons in the corpus callosum at birth are withdrawn during the first six months of postnatal development. I say withdrawn because neuron death in that period is fairly low; the 70 percent figure surely represents the withdrawal or pruning of some of the branches of a neuron's axon, not the death of the entire treelike neuron.

And what neurons are these, anyway, that send their axons over such long distances between hemispheres and front to back within a hemisphere? The major pipelines for long corticocorticals, such as the arcuate fasciculus connecting temporal and frontal 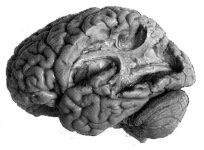 lobes, have long been noted. But there are also spotty projections, discovered a half-century ago in the days of strychnine neuronography. They are quite widespread and modern neuroanatomical techniques have revealed that they may be organized into macrocolumns and layers. So what are the pipeline and spotty long-distance projections doing? Surely they are biasing the distant basins of attraction, at a minimum. But might they clone hexagons like a *faux* fax?

THERE ARE TWO TYPES OF CORTICOCORTICAL projections, those that stay within the cortical layers and those that loop down through the white matter. The former, which are the intrinsic horizontal connections of the earlier chapters, are mostly local (though that can mean a few millimeters). The latter can go long distances, as from one hemisphere to another through the corpus callosum, though most only make a U-shaped passage through the white matter of one gyrus and then terminate in a nonadjacent patch of cortex that's only a few centimeters away.

All of those axons can come from one of the superficial pyramidal neurons we have been discussing. The long axons taking the white-matter routes typically terminate (though not exclusively) in the same superficial layers, once they arrive in distant cortex. So far, we've been looking at the ramifications of their axon branches that run *sideways* within layers 2 and 3, without ever looping through the white matter. These sidestepping connections are perhaps analogous to internal phone calls to neighboring offices, the U-axons to local calls within the city, and the lengthy U's to long distance calls.

Some cortical areas might be what Damasio calls convergence zones, a focal point for disparate modalities. I think of a convergence zone as something like the long-distance operator that sets up conference telephone calls, serving as the center of a funnel that rebroadcasts. Of course, the linkage could be centerless, as when a conference call of a half-dozen committee members is achieved by chaining, each person using their second phone line to link yet another member to the conversation via their phone's conference button.

The analogy to the telephone network may be misleading, both because of the phone system's point-to-point nature and because of the way open connections are established and maintained until hangup. Packet-based networks demonstrate an alternative, as when web pages are displayed and manipulated on the client machine without further attention from the server or the intervening network. We tend to think of those long cortico-cortical axon bundles as if they were fiber optic bundles that convey an image by thousands of little light pipes.

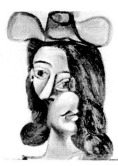 Of course, light pipes can go astray if the bundle is not carefully assembled; manufacturers have to make sure that neighbors at the sending end remain neighbors at the receiving end. An incoherent fiber bundle can create displaced facial features à la Picasso and neural wiring surely has many such imperfections.

And the fanout of connections at the far end (p. 19) is most unlike optical fiber terminations in another, more serious, way. A given axon fans out to connect with dozens of recipients, scattered over the better part of a millimeter. Such a point-to-area mapping, in the manner of a flashlight beam, only makes matters worse for any point-to-point mapping.

So, at first glimpse, it appears that corticocortical bundles are considerably worse than those incoherent fiber optic bundles that are factory rejects — unless, of course, something else is going on, not captured by our technological analogies to fax machines and fiber optics. Indeed, triangular arrays give one a different perspective on the fanout "problem" — even converting it into a virtue.

Suppose two adjacent members of the same triangular array send, in addition to their local axon branches, an axon via the white matter that terminates in a spray of terminals in the homologous area.

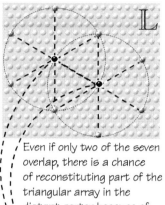

Even if only two of the seven overlap, there is a chance of reconstituting part of the triangular array in the distant cortex because of their synchronous EPSPs.

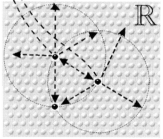

The off-target axons only provide a background noise against which the synchrony stands out. Since many members of the original triangular array may be contributing to coincidences, the seemingly diffuse many-to-many projections may nonetheless be capable of reconstituting an array. Enough such arrays, and the original spatiotemporal pattern in the hexagon is recreated as well, in a manner like error correcting codes.

HEXAGONAL CLONING with error-correction standardization could also happen in the target cortex, reproducing the spatiotemporal pattern that is being maintained on the sending end. I don't mean that in the sense of video point-to-point mapping, but rather in the sense of reconstituting the "weave" of the fabric without mimicking the extent of the fabric swatch (that dynamically changing patch on the quilt). In this scheme, you don't reconstitute the whole choir but a lesser number of singers, yet they're singing the same song and may themselves recruit neighbors to form another choir. Perhaps even a larger one.

We need to start with one note of that melody and its triangular array, indeed, with only one of its synchronized cells. There currently isn't data on the distant terminal fanout of one axon, nothing comparable in detail to that for the point-to-annulus fanout of the close-in branches, with the silent gaps described in chapter 2. We know that distant-terminal fanout exists, spanning macrocolumnar dimensions, but not much more. So I had to make a theoretician's assumption about the long-distance-call termination: that is, on average, a point-to-annulus fanout, just like the one back home in the 0.5 mm around the parent neuron (or minicolumn, p. 42) that structures the short path sidestepping. It's like a flashlight beam with a central bright spot, plus a bright peripheral ring.

That little assumption buys quite a lot compared to the point-to-area alternative.

Any one point in the target cortex is going to get inputs from a number of points in the sending cortex. How many? It might get one from the homologous point back home, directly on target for a point-to-point mapping. But there is also an active triangular array back home, all firing in synchrony. So the same point in target cortex might get another input from the fanout of axons from an adjacent point in the sending triangular array. Indeed, six such triangular nodes back home could make contact with the distant point in this manner, for a total of seven synchronous inputs — if nothing is lost along the way.

Let us say that half the potential axon terminals are lost. Still, it may only take a few synchronous inputs to recruit a neuron, given enough repetition. If the same thing happens 0.5 mm away, the pair can get their own triangular array going. Temporal dispersion may be less of a problem, as well. The synchrony criterion allows for a fair amount of time shift between the two arrivals; temporal summation of inputs depends on the decay times of the PSPs, and a few milliseconds dispersion might not matter very much. The terminals in the superficial layers suggest that NMDA mechanisms are involved and, given all the repetition to clean out the Mg^{++} plugs in the NMDA channels (p. 32), repeated pairing (at least at room temperature, the reoccupation of the NMDA channels by Mg^{++} requires tens or hundreds of milliseconds) might help recruit a target neuron into firing in near-synchrony with its distant "parents."

Even allowing for a fair amount of imprecise topographic mapping and a certain amount of temporal dispersion along the way, I think that a large enough sending area can get a small territory of similar arrays going in the target cortex (except, perhaps, for a change in the "0.5 mm" metric to reflect that typical of the target cortex). Error correction can shape up a standard version of the one-note triangular array in the distant cortex. If that happens for many of the triangular arrays, the spatiotemporal pattern at the target cortex is likely to be close to the tune playing back home.

The distant terminals might also prove to have the second annular ring of fanout branches as seen back home at twice the local metric distance; that would provide another six possible synchronized inputs. Only a few of the thirteen could suffice to start up a repeater node; only two such adjacent repeaters could suffice to start a local triangular array that can extend itself.

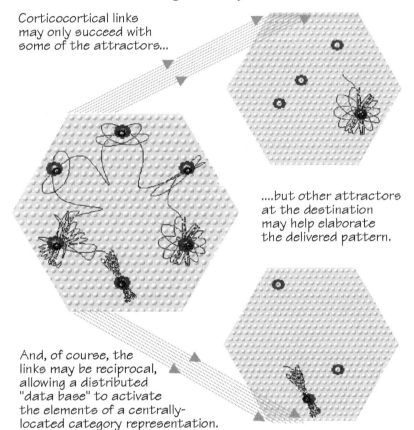

Corticocortical links may only succeed with some of the attractors...

....but other attractors at the destination may help elaborate the delivered pattern.

And, of course, the links may be reciprocal, allowing a distributed "data base" to activate the elements of a centrally-located category representation.

The strays will, of course, provide a certain amount of background noise. They might fog the pattern (p. 107) but there are two ways of getting around that. First, just as the view from two eyes separated by a few centimeters can disambiguate scenes that are too noisy for one eye alone, so we are bringing to bear a half-dozen or more elements of the sending array, all converging on a point. Second, I suspect the local automatic gain controls (p. 77) can allow the synchronous to be seen to the exclusion of the incoherent. Imagine a sea with islands standing out atop its surface. As error correction begins to operate locally, their positioning is sharpened up into a triangular array. As the AGC raises the sea level, the potentially fogging incoherent responses are submerged.

So, we have created a distant repeater of the triangular array back home. And that applies to each of the triangular arrays there, each interested in different features of an input (or contributing to different aspects of an output).

We have cloned the hexagon in distant cortex, the *faux* fax at last. And it is just the type of mechanism needed for linking together distributed features of a database, the question raised in chapter 7.

TWO ADJACENT HEXAGONS, once started up in the distant cortex and singing the same music, are sufficient to clone a choir producing the same melody, but success will depend on the exotic (literally, in another place) resonances. This spatiotemporal pattern's relative success in cloning competitions ought to depend on the same *types* of factors as in the sending cortex: biases to the local basins of attraction.

But they ought to differ in detail, to arrive against a different set of resonances, biased by different ratio of neuromodulators — and so the competitive outcome could be very different than back home. Just as emigrants may thrive in distant places, so *faux* faxed spatiotemporal patterns might find a completely different reception in the distant cortex. Typically, of course, dying out without issue, but occasionally thriving.

Not all of the parent attractors may arrive intact; even when they do, they arrive against a very different background of passive attractors than existed back home, both from short-term and long-term memories residing in the target hexagons. Furthermore, there may be several *faux* faxes arriving at the same time from different senders — which means we have a new form of competition, quite in addition to the side-by-side dog and cat pavers type of lateral competition for space introduced in chapter 4.

For all these reasons, the spatiotemporal patterns in the target region may not be mere superpositions of the contributors, those jazz performance overlays. In Hebb's other dual trace memory system, you can get melding of attractors in "bilingual belts" from noncontemporaneous occupations of the target area. Such exotic combinations are best introduced, probably to no one's surprise, after a preliminary reminder about sex.

AMONG THE ACCELERATORS OF EVOLUTION IS SEX, both in the sense of recombination but also in Darwin's sense of sexual selection serving to create elaborate peacock tails much more quickly than environmental selection would ever do. Among all our dichotomies, is there anything that could be analogous to sex?

The novel aspect of the biological invention of sex was not the exchange of genetic material (bacterial conjugation and retroviruses had likely been busy doing that for some time) but the development of more specialized vehicles called gametes that had storehouses of energy, handy for either mobility or fetal development. And the interesting thing about gametes is that equal-sized ones weren't stable; once there were slight variants in stored metabolic energy, evolutionarily stable strategy considerations took them to the extremes of little sperm and big ova. This gamete dimorphism is what gives rise to most of the secondary characteristics of males and females, including their differing reproductive strategies.

Because sperm are cheap (an adult human male may produce 40 million *a day*), one male has the potential of fathering an almost unlimited number of offspring. Ova are expensive and so one female has a more limited number of potential offspring (a human female is born with her *lifetime* supply of a few hundred, which is still an order of magnitude more than she can possibly rear). On the other hand, a female is almost guaranteed some offspring, at least in comparison to a male who may well get none at all because of the competition for access to females. In many species, this leads to females being choosy about sexual partners at the same time that males are more indiscriminate.

Female choice can drive sexual selection; she might prefer long, shiny feathers. Male competition (excluding other males is the name of the game in harem-style mating systems) selects for variants in testosterone production. This can lead to male gorillas twice the size of females; female choice is carried to extremes in peacocks (though perhaps starting with feathers indicating a male's health or genes for resistance to parasites, the simple-minded *more-is-better* criterion repeated over and over).

To ask if such kinds of sexual selection could be going on in a system such as neocortical hexagonal competitions, it is not necessary to identify a traditional male/female distinction. For example, a simple and a complex code, with a tendency to merge, might suffice. So long as there are at least two general types of codes, differing in some inheritable property that affects reproduction, one can have something like sexual selection operating.

Cloning opportunities abound for spatiotemporal patterns in neocortex, but the major simple-complex dichotomy so far has been short single-note melodies versus long chorded stanzas. Neural pattern complexity is obviously a continuum — but so, too, was gamete energy investment, at first sight. Might there be the same tendency to go to extremes because intermediates tend to be outcompeted?

Get used to thinking that there is nothing Nature loves so well as to change existing forms and to make new ones like them.
MARCUS AURELIUS, *Meditations*

One set of extremes was seen in the chapter 7 analogy to the hash versus the full text, where mere recognition can be done cheaply (hash the incoming and compare it with a low-dimensional database of hashes of the higher-dimensional stored memories), but recall is more demanding, requiring an expensive investment in reconstructing detail (probably starting with an intermediate representation, the prototype or some other form of loose-fitting abstract). Still, complex spatiotemporal patterns (up to the size that can still be contained in a hexagon) can clone, just as simple ones can.

But the production of new individuals (as opposed to just another clone) can involve both error and recombination. Is there any possible sexlike dichotomy in recombination? We now have three types of superposition: those "in-house" ones associated with the intrinsic horizontals and borderline superpositions, the "local call" ones associated with U-fiber projections within a cortical area (and often within a particular sensory modality), and the "long distance" ones where different sensory and motor modalities may converge. We also have several superposition mechanisms, the active ephemeral ones and the new attractors in the connectivity that might blend experiences from different times and places in belts of overlap.

SUPERIMPOSING TWO STANZAS is perhaps more difficult than adding a simple trill to an existing stanza. Superimposing a complex spatiotemporal pattern upon another complex one, in such a way that it can be embedded in the connectivity and later reconstituted, is surely a more difficult task than successfully superimposing two simples or superimposing a simple on a complex.

In biology, there is always the issue of the recombination's viability. Most are unsuccessful in reaching reproductive age, whether from juvenile mortality or (as naturally happens with 80 percent of human conceptions) spontaneous abortion. Matings between related species can occasionally produce hybrids, though many are dead ends because of sterility. So, too, we have compatibility issues when dealing with a hexagonal connectivity that simultaneously supports many different basins of attraction: some superimposed spatiotemporal patterns are going to be captured by the existing attractors, others are going to fail to be incorporated, but a few might successfully change some aspect of the hexagon's repertoire (likely only a trills' worth of one of its many melodies) via a connectivity alteration.

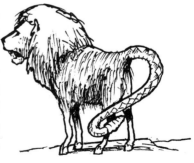

Chimeras, as in the she-monster of Greek mythology that had the head of a lion, the body of a goat, and the tail of a snake, are considerably more rare than hybrids. Still, occasionally an individual is seen with odd features such as two blood types that suggest fraternal twin fetuses amalgamated into one individual early in gestation, or that a mother gained some cells from a gestating fetus. One can imagine similar amalgamations of attractor basins, just as in those Charles Ives melodies with an intruded snippet of *Yankee Doodle*. Though copied everywhere, such an intrusion might have meaning in only one cortical area, just as only part of the genome is decoded by the specialized cells of the liver but all are copied during mitosis there.

The recombination issue could be avoided, of course, if the connectivity were a tabula rasa: so plastic that the hexagonal mosaic became a buffer, holding only one very detailed attractor in its connectivity (and not dozens). Intermediate levels of plasticity might allow multiple melodies from the same connectivity, or they might allow anything more than a week old to be overwritten. But one can imagine a hexagon's worth of connectivity that added attractor lobes only reluctantly, and only to some of its dozens of separate attractors. That would mean that simple-complex pairings would be the most common "new individuals," loosely analogous to the way sexual reproduction forms new individuals by recombining a small and a large gamete.

Tacking on an additional feature creates, of course, an *extra-strange attractor* (given that attractors with multiple lobes were originally called strange attractors, as in the two-lobe butterfly attractor). This makes our hint of sex in convergence zones extra strange.

BUT THIS NEW INDIVIDUAL ISN'T DOUBLY STRANGE: it doesn't carry around nearly equal numbers of contributions from both parents in the familiar heterozygous manner, with two alleles often available. Think of the offspring as very much like one parent (indeed, it *is* that parent, modified — but since the parent exists in numerous hexagonal clones, and only a few may be modified, the parent pattern may live on elsewhere), with just a touch here and there of the other parent.

What the new individual has, rather than all those alternative alleles of the truly heterozygous, may be a working link to the minor parent: the umbilical cord hasn't been broken. That trill's worth of addition could be the hash that, elsewhere in neocortex under some circumstances, evokes a full-text spatiotemporal pattern and sends it back. The new individual could inherit from its major parent a whole collection of such links to outlying hexagons and their more detailed attractors. So here we have not only a candidate for what integrates the sight-sound-feel-pronunciation of *comb* but a suggestion of how we might tack on a new attribute (those broken teeth that help identify it as *my* comb!) with a trill-like link.

One can imagine reciprocal connections or strange attractors that work too well, as when a stimulus in one sensory modality evokes a strong memory in another (an element of the condition known as synesthesia). Links that fail could presumably give rise to a variety of minor (anomia) and major (agnosia) complaints, simply from the failure to make accustomed links.

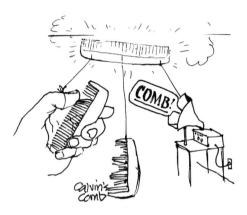

An attractor's complexity may, or may not, be expensive to create (simple rules can have complex consequences), but it is surely expensive to maintain over a long haul, simply from what economists would call opportunity costs (in this case, lost opportunities, foregone options in the name of persistence or stability). No matter how large your hard disk, it rapidly fills up; surely your brain has the same accretion problem, even in childhood. Maintaining attractors has a cost, commonly noticed as lengthening access times that slow performance at some tasks (a subject to be addressed later, at p.185).

CONCRETE THINKING provides one example of premature closure, of terminating a search for mental links too soon. And we can now see one way in which this could happen: with a different plurality for successful links than for successful closure.

The simplest model for closure is the movement choice example of chapter 4 (p. 57), where various candidates for a hand movement competed until some plurality was reached, at which subcortical mechanisms launched the movement with the strongest chorus. Call this plurality requirement the N for action, N_a. Activating the kth link out of this same territory takes N_k to get the same spatiotemporal pattern going with smaller numbers in the target cortex.

Suppose closure for action normally takes a chorus of 100 hexagons, while establishing a link only takes 50. Then suppose that N_a is lowered to 40 without changing the linkage requirements, or that the N_k requirements were raised to 125 because of signal/noise ratio problems at the destination. In either case, you would act without considering some of the linked attractors stored elsewhere. And so you would have trouble seeing analogies. In extreme cases, you might even dissociate the various sensory representations of the same object, as in the agnosias.

The half-second-and-longer reaction times seen in much cognitive processing have always been a puzzle from the standpoint of conduction times and synaptic delays, all an order of magnitude briefer. Add to the time to recruit a local chorus the time needed to form a second territory via a link, and cross-modality matching experiments might require the better part of a second, simply because of the repetitions needed to gradually develop the links.

With a darwinian process operating in cerebral cortex, you can now imagine how stratified stability could generate a strata of concepts that are inexpressible, except by roundabout, inadequate means — as when we know things of which we cannot speak. Decomposing them via successive links into speakable concepts is a lot of additional work beyond that point at which you sense the problem's criteria have been fulfilled.

CORTICOCORTICAL IMPROVEMENTS are an interesting issue here, as surely the corticocortical axons do something simpler most of the time, not arbitrary spatiotemporal patterns.

The axon fanout at the destination, if not tuned up for recreating triangular arrays, presumably produces a distorted version of the spatiotemporal pattern at the origin. Presumably the receiving cortex handles this in the manner of categorical perception, tuning up to recognize special cases. When the number of vocabulary items is dozens to hundreds, this probably suffices.

We, however, have vocabularies of 10^5 and can extend them to novel concepts, such as when we talk about how many angels can dance on the head of a pin. That suggests we have improved our corticocorticals to the point that they can transmit arbitrary spatiotemporal patterns. I will discuss this again at the end of the final chapter, when I engage in a brief digression into Universal Grammar, but here I wish to point out the route to improving corticocorticals from special-case codes to arbitrary codes.

> Assuming a Darwin Machine already exists on both ends, then the size of the sending array could be a major determinant of whether the origin's spatiotemporal pattern could be recreated at the destination.
>
> If the axon fanout is not sufficiently point-to-annulus, then additional point-to-area inhibition at the destination could help develop it.
>
> If the axon fanout is normally pruned far back during pre- and post-natal development, then neoteny might help conserve the fanout until Darwin Machine activity began exercising it.

LONG-DISTANCE CONNECTIONS, one is tempted to claim, are something like an extended family. If an area's local history of cloning competitions serves to create a community of interacting individuals, then the long-distance links are something like the scientific community in the early days of the Royal Society, that interacted mostly by letters with many copies, and later, publications.

Or like the virtual communities of cyberspace. Such interacting groups don't have all the features of local communities — you can't, for instance, borrow a cup of sugar from the neighbors. But then you don't have to listen to the neighbor's barking dog, either.

[A critical approach to education] is based on evolutionary epistemology, which claims that we never receive knowledge, but rather create it; we create it by modifying the knowledge we already have; and we modify our existing knowledge only when we uncover inadequacies in it that we had not recognized heretofore. Accepting this as an explanation of how knowledge grows, I have suggested that teachers construe their roles as facilitators of the growth of their students' knowledge.

HENRY PERKINSON, 1993

It used to be supposed that the world is just out there, on the other side of a clear sensory window pane. Now we're sure that the experienced world is itself a construct, a somewhat unstable patchwork of mental models driven partly by what's outside, partly by genetically ordained internal grammars, partly by the local cultural templates we imbibe from childhood on (including the language we use to categorize and communicate our grasp of the world). It's naive to suppose that culture and language capture "just how things are," and hence to fear and hate anyone whose inner maps conflict with our own, but still it takes quite an effort to see that our worlds are built up in accord with these internal maps or theories.

DAMIEN BRODERICK, 1996

9

Chimes on
the Quarter Hour

A script is a structure that describes appropriate
sequences of events in a particular context. A script is
made up of slots and requirements about what can fill
those slots. The structure is an interconnected whole,
and what is in one slot affects what can be in another.
Scripts handle stylized everyday situations. They are
not subject to much change, nor do they provide the
apparatus for handling totally novel situations. Thus, a
script is a predetermined, stereotyped sequence of
actions that defines a well-known situation.

ROGER SHANK and ROBERT ABELSON, 1977

W E HAVE AN URGE, ALMOST A COMPULSION, to finish a
well-known sequence. Recall how a crying child can
be distracted, by singing a familiar nursery rhyme and
then prompting the child to fill in the last word of the line. This
is so compulsive a response that it often overrides the child's
crying and eventually stops it.

We create sequences when we speak a sentence that we've
never spoken before, or improvise at jazz, or plan a career. We
invent dance steps. Even as four-year-olds, we can play roles,
achieving a level of abstraction not seen in even the smartest apes.
Many of our beyond-the-apes behaviors involve novel strings of
behaviors, often compounded: phonemes chunked into words,
words into word phrases, and (as in this paragraph) word phrases
into complicated sentences with nested ideas.

Rules for made-up games illustrate the memory aspect of this novelty: we must judge possible moves against serial-order rules, for example, in solitaire where you must alternate colors as you place cards in descending order. Preschool children will even make up such arbitrary rules, and then judge possible actions against them. We abandon many of the possible moves that we consider in a card game, once we check them out against our serial-order memories of the rules. In shaping up a novel sentence to speak, we are checking our candidate word strings against overlearned ordering rules that we call syntax and grammar. We even memorize unique sequential episodes without intending to do so: when you try to remember where you lost your keys, the various places that you visited since you last used a key can often be recalled.

> Narrative is one of the ways in which we speak, one of the large categories in which we think. Plot is its thread of design and its active shaping force, the product of our refusal to allow temporality to be meaningless, our stubborn insistence on making meaning in the world and in our lives.
>
> PETER BROOKS, 1984

THERE IS A GREAT DEAL OF INFORMATION hidden in the overall flow of even nonsense words, presumably the reason why we appreciate Charles Dodgson's youthful poem, "'Twas brillig, and the slithy toves/Did gyre and gimble in the wabe; All mimsy were the borogoves/ And the mome raths outgrabe."

Sequential form alone, with even less hint of meaning, can be sufficient to bring forward a complete phrase from memory. Sometimes we can do this from what initially appears totally

Freunde, Römer, Mitbürger, gebt mir Gehör! Ich komme, Cäsars Leiche zu bestatten, nicht, ihn zu loben.

incomprehensible (I am indebted to Dan Dennett for this lovely example of just-sufficient disguise).

Now even if you only know a few words of this language, and have never seen the faded, centuries-old font and the spellings of the time, you can probably recognize this quotation within a few minutes. That is, you can *recognize* that it's familiar but you can't *recall* it in detail without a lot more effort. But once you do recall it, and its short-form name, X, it will become so obvious that it will be difficult to look back and see it as anything other than X (that's because your X attractor has been activated, firmly capturing variants).

We're used to the idea that we can pop out hidden objects from fragments, but to recognize something far less familiar, and only from the general form of the sentence (and perhaps the cadence, if mumbled subvocally), shows how much information is contained in the form of a long string. Extreme cases such as Dennett's illustrate our exquisite capability for serial-ordered forms that are presumably utilized, in more rigid fashion, by scripts – and, of course, more generally and abstractly by music.

In trying to comprehend a sentence, we often seek out missing information because of encountering a word that must connect with certain other portions of the string. I discuss this in chapter 5 of *How Brains Think* as part of linguistic argument structure: a verb such as *give* requires three nouns to fill the roles of actor, recipient, and object given. When you encounter *give*, you go searching for all three nouns or noun phrases. One now sees billboard advertising slogans that read *Give him.* We easily infer "you" as the implied actor but the still-incomplete sentence sends us off on a compulsive search for the object to be given (this is a technique to make the ad more memorable by increasing dwell duration).

Can hexagonal cloning competitions help us appreciate the underpinnings of these abilities to string things together? And the search for the missing segment?

STATE MACHINES ARE THE TRADITIONAL MODEL for sequencing and stage setting. The Barcelona subway, for example, has ticket machines that require me to first select the ticket type, then the number of passengers, then deposit the coins, then retrieve the ticket. The successful completion of one state causes the machine to advance to its next state (though it times out if I spend too much time fumbling for the correct coins). Barcelona even has an automata museum devoted to nineteenth-century state machines and robots. State machines are often easy to build but difficult to operate intuitively (just think of programming your videotape recorder).

Might switching gaits of locomotion involve a state machine? Note that jog or lope is not required as an intermediate gait between walk and run; the system can make transitions in various orders, suggesting that it is not a simple state machine. Still, stage-setting remains an important possibility for advancing a chain of thought or action.

Chimes on the quarter hour were easily heard from my hotel balcony in Barcelona, the local church reminding me that time flies — and that I write too slowly. Such chimes are the most familiar example of combining spatiotemporal pattern and state machine. American grandfather clocks, such as the one my father once con-structed, use a slightly different tune on the

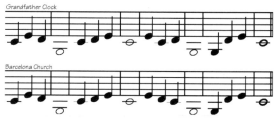

three-quarter hour. I have persuaded my mother to write out the corresponding musical notes that adorn this chapter (I can read music but not write it down, another example of recall being more difficult than recognition, of production being more difficult than understanding).

SPATIOTEMPORAL PATTERNS WITHIN THE HEXAGON are, so far, my model for an activated cerebral code — not only for objects and events but for composites such as categories. For the stored code, it's the spatial-only patterning of synaptic connections that give rise to basins of attraction. Resurrection of a complex spatio-temporal pattern might involve changing from one attractor to another. Adding on another attractor might, on the chaotic itinerancy model, be like adding another city to the traveling salesman's route.

Because the hexagon's spatiotemporal pattern is mappable to a musical scale, thanks to having similar numbers of elements, I have talked of this spatiotemporal pattern as like a line of music; even timeless objects such as Kant's triangles still have a temporal aspect to their code in my theory. Note how much temporal patterning increases the coding space over chord combinations alone, even if time were only to be sliced into 64 segments: each point in the hexagon now has 64 possible states.

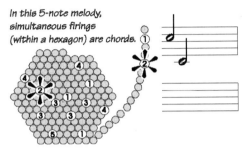

In this 5-note melody, simultaneous firings (within a hexagon) are chords.

But because some of the things we memorize are themselves extended in time, we have to consider whether the category code is strung out in distinct spatiotemporal units, like the frames of movie film. We involuntarily memorize brief episodes (though not very accurately). On the movement side, we produce motor outputs that chain together unitary actions, as when we unlock a door or dial a telephone. Asleep, we create narratives with improbable qualities that are often signaled by nonsensical segues and juxtapositions (nonviable chimeras, as it were).

Is the sequence's representation simply a chain of elementary spatiotemporal patterns, skillfully segued like a medley of songs? Or is neural sequencing more complicated, like those mental models that intervene when recalling a text? Certainly phonemics suggests some obligatory stage-setting (one reason that mechanical text-to-speech conversion is complicated is that look-ahead is required: some phonemes are modified when followed by certain other ones, so a planning buffer is needed).

Just as in biology, there are two levels of mechanism to consider here: active firing and those passive bumps and ruts in the road. Active firing, as we have seen, is especially important for cloning spatiotemporal patterns; the territory attained may be important both locally and in seeding the *faux* fax distant version. And, of course, it may modify the connectivity beneath it.

But how does a sequence get started from the passive connectivity and elaborate itself into extended lines of "music"? Is this the activation of a multilobed attractor within a single hexagon, or a circuit rider visiting different hexagons, each of whom contribute a segment? Like the recognition-recall problem, we may have another multi-level solution — a hash could serve as a fingerprint for a full text, or a loose-fitting, centrally-located abstract could have links to outlying details. In the manner of the multimodality funnel for *comb*, recall might be a matter of links but with activation in a certain order contributed by a multilobed attractor in the temporal equivalent of a convergence zone, acting much like the orchestral conductor in adjusting startup times.

ONE CLUE TO SEQUENCE REPRESENTATION is that we are often able to decompose them at will, for both sensory and movement sequences. We easily discard the first three words of "Repeat after me — I swear to tell. . . ." when replying. Compare that to the rat that thinks life is more complicated than it really is, circling three times before pressing the bar in the Skinner box, simply because that's what he happened to have done prior to being rewarded for some prior bar press (shaping rats out of superstitious behavior is an important bit of customization of experiments to individual subjects).

We can discard the inefficient parts of an exploratory sequence when repeating it, just as speakers can often paraphrase long questions from the audience before answering them. Indeed, our memories seem organized this way: readers tend to remember the mental model they constructed from a text, rather than the text itself, and such abstraction probably happens as well for "film-clip experiences," such as being an eyewitness to an accident.

Some complicated sequences can, with enough practice, become securely enough embedded to survive major insults to the brain, for example, the aphasic patient who can sing the national anthem, even though he cannot speak a nonroutine sentence, one that requires customizing a sequence before actually speaking. It's not that different from what happens in all of us, normally. A dart throw or basketball free throw, where the object is to do the movement exactly the same each time by getting "in the groove" appropriate to the standard distance and standard projectile, may be secure — at least, when compared to throwing at novel targets. Novelty may require a lot of offline planning during get-set, customizing the command sequence for the particular situation.

THE DIFFICULTY OF THROWING ACCURATELY is actually what attracted me into postulating that spatiotemporal patterns were cloned in the brain (to conclude the history in chapter 6), long before any of the detailed physiological studies of throwing performance. In the summer of 1980, I was sitting on a beach in the San Juan Islands, looking out the Strait of Juan de Fuca between Washington State and British Columbia, and throwing stones at a rock that I had placed atop a log. I seldom hit it, so I moved closer and finally starting hitting it more frequently.

I got to thinking about why the task seemed so difficult. It was, I realized, that there was a launch window. If I let loose of my projectile too early, before the launch window was reached, the projectile arched too high and went too far. If I let loose too late, the path was too straight and hit below the target. If I moved closer, or used a larger target, the launch window lasted longer and so was easier to attain. Elementary physics. My motor neurons, I reflected, were too noisy — and so couldn't settle down to controlling projectile release precisely enough to stay within the launch window.

That's where the story, hardly worth retelling, would surely have ended — except that I just happened to have some knowledge about how jittery the spinal motor neurons were. Indeed, I had done my Ph.D. thesis on that very subject 14 years earlier. So how wide was the launch window, in milliseconds? Does it match up with the noise levels of typical motor neurons?

On the ferry ride home, I assumed it was just a matter of looking up the right formula in my old physics textbooks (I had, after all, been a physics major). But as soon as I thumbed through both my elementary and advanced mechanics texts, I realized that the variables of target size, height of release point above target, and the possible range of velocities meant that I was going to need to derive an appropriate equation from basic Newtonian principles. So I customized an equation, reveling in the fact that my rusty calculus still worked. And realizing that few things in biology could be similarly derived from basic principles, that particular histories were all important in a way that they weren't in physics.

For throwing at a rabbit-sized target (10 cm high, 20 cm deep) from about a car length away (4 meters), the launch windows averaged out at about 11 milliseconds wide. That was also about what I figured was the inherent noise in single motor neurons while in their self-paced mode.

Yes, they matched — but I realized that something was very wrong. Most of us, I supposed, could hit that rabbit-sized target from two car lengths, or even three. The launch window for 8 meter throws worked out to 1.4 milliseconds. And there was no way that the motor neurons I knew so well were ever likely to attain that. I couldn't consult the experts — I *was* the expert (at least on cat motor neurons, where the most detailed work had been done, and I knew that human forearm motor neurons weren't much better from the neurologists's EMG recordings).

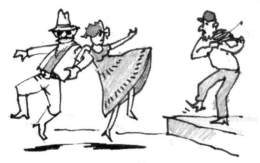

Perhaps, you might say (as I eventually did) that the spinal motor neurons are simply being commanded to fire at the right time by descending commands from motor cortex — that is, not making the decisions within those basins of attraction in spinal cord itself. The spinal motor neurons might be noisy on their own but, with the brain serving as a square-dance caller, they might be precise repeaters. The precision might be upstream.

That, too, should have been the end of the story. But I'd done a study only five years earlier on motor cortex neurons. And those cortical neurons were much noisier than spinal motor neurons under similar conditions, not quieter. No escape there. I'd been talking informally to neurophysiologists who worked in other brain centers, regarding the possibility of accurate "clocks," and it didn't look as if anywhere in the brain had superprecise neurons that ticked along with very little timing jitter.

So I had a persisting theoretical puzzle to chew on: how did we get precision timing from relatively jittery neurons? Salvation arrived in the form of a reprint that crossed my desk shortly thereafter, delayed for about one year by the Italian postal system and slow boats. It in turn led me to a lovely paper by John Clay and Bob DeHaan in the *Biophysical Journal*, about chick heart cells in a culture dish. Each cell, when sitting in isolation, was beating irregularly. If they nudged two cells together, their beats would synchronize. If they kept adding cells, the jitter declined with each additional cell added to the cluster; what sounded as irregular as rain on the roof became as regular as a steadily dripping faucet.

The interval's coefficient of variation fell as the inverse square root of N. To halve the interbeat jitter, just quadruple the number of cells in the cluster. And it wasn't just pacemaker cells but many kinds of relaxation oscillator, as J. T. Enright's 1980 *Science* paper (subtitled "A reliable neuronal clock from unreliable components?") soon made clear.

All it took to throw with precision, I concluded, was lots of clones of the movement commands from the brain, all singing the same spatiotemporal pattern in a chorus. But the numbers of cells required were staggering: to double your throwing distance, while maintaining the same hit rate, required recruiting a chorus 64 times larger than the original one. Tripling the target distance took 729 times as many. Clearly, the four-fold increase in neocortical numbers during ape-to-human evolution wasn't enough to handle this, as I'd hoped; those extra neurons would have to be temporarily borrowed somehow, perhaps in the way that the expert choir borrows the inexpert audience when singing the *Hallelujah Chorus*.

Paradoxically, the Law of Large Numbers effectively said that the nonexperts could actually help improve performance, beyond that of the experts alone. It took me another decade to imagine a way of recruiting the larger chorus: that cloning mechanism for spatiotemporal patterns of *Act I*.

APROPOS THE ADVANTAGES OF NON-EXPERTS, the composer Brian Eno tells an interesting story about an orchestra whose members were, quite intentionally, a mixture of the mildly experienced and the self-selected musically naive. In recounting his experience with the Portsmouth Symphonia, Eno said that one would occasionally hear some nimble playing emerge from the too-early, too-loud, off-tune chaos — which he called "classical music reduced to some sort of statistical average."

Some amateur-night variation is very much what I imagine first happening in our premotor cortex as one "gets set" to throw at a novel target: that the variants gradually standardize to become the chorus. I imagine the practiced precision appearing in the several seconds that it takes hexagonal competition and error-correction to stabilize a widespread precision version of the most successful variant.

THE CD PLAYER OR JUKEBOX on automatic serves as a fancier-than-chimes example of a state machine for spatiotemporal patterns, pulling in one platter after another and playing them. Like chimes on the quarter hour, this suggests separate performances that don't overlap in time, in the manner of the various instrument groups that perform one after the other at the beginning of *A Young Person's Guide to the Orchestra*.

One can, with such circuit-riding state machine analogies, easily imagine how the compulsion to finish a song line could arise in those crying children. What's being stirred up is that central state machine with links to the components. As each is activated, feedback from it reinforces the forward motion of the state machine attractor. The prompting voice advances it too, and the omission of the prompt on the last word may not matter, once the

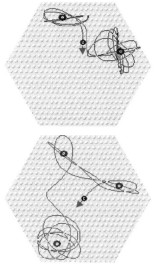

Path of pendulum attracted by two magnets, shown superimposed on a hexagon, with bifurcation to a second attractor.

Adding third attractor

endogenous attractor has generated sufficient forward moment-
um.

One (likely oversimplified) model of schemas for sequence is
quite similar. A hexagonal code for the calling sequence itself is
likely a multilobed attractor, one that cycles through its various
basins of attraction and, in the manner of an orchestra's
conductor, activates one link after another to outlying hexagonal
territories that generate their own spatiotemporal patterns. But
more typical sequencers are probably more like typical orchestral
compositions, where the conductor brings in a new group to
overlay the ongoing contributions of the earlier groups of
instruments. In a canon, a melody repeats after a delay to overlap
(as in "Row, Row, Row Your Boat"). There is, of course, no
requirement for a conductor per se; string quartets manage
without one, and complex patterns can arise from simple rules.

A more serious problem for the neurological imagination is
finding the missing nouns in
that *give* sentence. Sentences too
are sequences at the performance level (though not in underlying structure, where trees and
boxes-within-boxes are better
analogies than paths). Think of
give starting up an attractor with
three lobes, each with reinforcing feedback from its linked
attractor basins at a distance. It
may be that this central attract-
or's spatiotemporal pattern

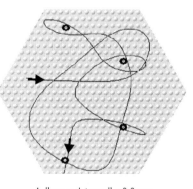

A "grand tour" of four
basins of attraction.

undergoes a characteristic change when all side basins have full
feedback: it changes from *unfulfilled* to *fulfilled* and this is one of
the necessary conditions for you to judge the sentence as making
sense. So long as it remains in condition *unfulfilled*, you keep
trying out different candidates for those actor-recipient-object
nouns. Actually, I assume that many variations exist in parallel,
and that they compete for territory until one achieves the
especially powerful *fulfilled* spatiotemporal pattern — in effect,
that particular variant shouts "Bingo!" because all its slots are

legally filled. (I discuss a *lingua ex machina* more explicitly in chapter 5 of *How Brains Think*).

BRIAN ENO ALSO NOTES that doing something well ("becoming a pro") can lead to a lack of alertness about interesting variations, as if (in my terms) an attractor had created a compelling groove. Fortunately, the neocortical Darwin Machine for orchestrating movements promises to not only be quicker (seconds vs. lifetimes) at producing pros, but also resettable so that amateurs alert to interesting variations can still occur a bit later in the same work space.

An internal model allows a system to look ahead to the
future consequences of current actions, without
actually committing itself to those actions. In
particular, the system can avoid acts that would set it
irretrievably down some road to future disaster
("stepping off a cliff"). Less dramatically, but equally
important, the model enables the agent to make
current "stage-setting" moves that set up later moves
that are obviously advantageous. The very essence of a
competitive advantage, whether it be in chess or
economics, is the discovery and execution of stage-
setting moves.

JOHN HOLLAND, 1992

10

The Making of Metaphor

When people think seriously, they think abstractly;
they conjure up simplified pictures of reality called
concepts, theories, models, paradigms. Without such
intellectual constructs, there is, William James said,
only "a bloomin' buzzin' confusion."

SAMUEL P. HUNTINGTON, 1993

KANT SAID THAT OUR METAPHORS comprise the conceptual spectacles through which we view the world. In part, that's surely a matter of our general tendency to borrow concepts and vocabulary, selecting them from elements of our more accessible physical and social worlds, and trying to apply them to reasoning and emotion. Sometimes we do it well, but at other times, we get trapped by inadequate metaphors, as when we try to propitiate the weather — as if it were a person, susceptible to bribes or flattery.

How we carve up our world depends on what's out there — and on the analogies we bring to bear. We often talk as if ideas and thoughts were objects, that words and sentences were containers for these objects, and that communication was simply a matter of finding the right object, packaging it up, and sending it to a recipient who unpacks it. We often talk of rational thought as if it were just the algorithmic manipulation of such symbols. We go looking for computational elements in the brain that could accomplish such logical operations with virtual objects. This, alas, leaves no room for guessing or imagination. Our inadequate container schemas have boxed us in.

160

[Edgar Allan Poe's *Eureka*] dismissed the methods of both Bacon and Aristotle as the paths to certain knowledge.... He argued for a third method to knowledge which he called imagination . . . . Imagination, or genius, or intuition, lets the classification start so that the successive iterations, back and forth between the empirical and the rational, hone the product until it finally conforms to nature. Only then is the dross of the classifier skimmed away and a true order in nature, if it exists, revealed.

ALLAN SANDAGE, 1995

Without imagination, we have no mechanisms by which to use reflection to mold experience, to bring something new out of the old, or to sympathetically project ourselves into someone else's shoes. There's no room, either, in traditional categories from set theory, as they box us in with necessary and sufficient conditions rather than allowing for fuzzy edges.

Most of us normally function at a level of description that regards a chair as an object rather than a collection of wood grains or molecules or atoms. We are comfortable talking about a chair, even if we are physicists. We're also comfortable talking about a schematic level of representation such as furniture. We use such abstractions to make sense of the common features of diverse experiences. Our borrowing from the physical and social worlds often aids feeling our way around, within a different level of organization.

If we are to have meaningful, connected experiences — ones that we can comprehend and reason about — we must be able to discern patterns to our actions, perceptions, and conceptions. Underlying our vast network of interrelated literal meanings (all of those words about objects and actions) are those imaginative structures of understanding such as schema and metaphor, such as the mental imagery that allows us to extrapolate a path, or zoom in on one part of the whole, or zoom out until the trees merge into a forest. Can such properties be represented by the aforementioned cerebral codes and darwinian processes?

Thinking is a process by which some pattern is actualized from the intentional structure into meaning and deployed into the world. Thoughts differ from meanings in being the fleeting, unstable, dynamic operants by which meanings are constructed and carried. They enact the emergence of meaning as a set of relations in a place in an intentional structure, in accordance with which representations are shaped by action into the world. A representation formed and sent by one brain evoked thought that leads to the construction of meaning in a brain receiving the representation.

WALTER J. FREEMAN, 1995

ANY SCHEMATIC OUTLINE can be called a schema, but the latter term is more typically used for particularly common representations, not only for sensations but for movements as well. Though a schema is more abstract than a rich mental image of an object, it's grounded in our everyday experiences, often making reference to our own body moving through our daily world with its visual scene that streams past our head. One schema is UP-DOWN, a generalization of many experiences, as is the notion of a PATH.

Schemas are often about one thing relative to another. They include the little works of grammar — only a few dozen in number — that position things or events relative to each other on a mental map: relative location (*above, below, in, on, at, by, next to*), relative direction (*to, from, through, left, right, up, down*), relative time (*before, after, while*, and the various indicators of tense such as -*ed*), relative number (*many, few, some*, the -*s* of plurality), relative possibility (*can, may, might*), relative contingency (*unless, although, until, because*), possession (*of*, the possessive version of -*s, have*), agency (*by*), purpose (*for*), necessity (*must, have to*), obligation (*should, ought to*), existence (*be*), nonexistence (*no, none, not, un-*), and more.

Other common schemas are BLOCKAGE, CENTER-PERIPHERY, FULL-EMPTY, MORE-LESS, NEAR-FAR, SPLITTING, ATTRACTION, BALANCE, MATCHING, REMOVING A RESTRAINT, ATTRACTS, CIRCLES, PART-WHOLE, and the easy-to-misuse CONTAINMENT. Note that schemas tend to refer to movement, rather than static properties (they're often *structures* of an activity, not *attributes* of an object such as wet or cold). Even more than abstracts, schemas are flexible enough to fit many similar situations with differing details. They're few enough in number to be handled as special cases, just as the several hundred irregular verbs are handled as exceptions to the general rule for past tense, add -ed.

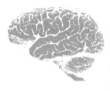 As chapter 7 discussed, hexagonal cerebral codes allow for forming new spatiotemporal patterns from several sources. Note that superpositions need not keep all of the component attractors; the category *Fruit* can amalgamate some the attractors from *Apple* and *Orange* into a new strange attractor. The same thing can happen in going from features such as *round* and *red* to an object-level description such as *Apple*. We don't have to amalgamate all the component's features into the category. The test is whether one can selectively reactivate the object-level codes from the higher category, whether one can get back from *Apple* to *red*.

There are two major ways in which categories could arise: from active superpositions of hexagonal codes and from linking them (as when the U-fibers copy a pattern into another cortical area with different attractors, as when recognition-only hashes or loose-fitting abstracts are elaborated into full-text spatiotemporal patterns). Both results are capable of representing dynamic aspects (spatiotemporal patterns can represent both static and dynamic things); both can accommodate malleable edges. They seem amenable to the fuzzy types of categories that we form up from prototypes, with less prototypical members at various distances from the category's center.

Prototypes (a good American English /i/ vowel, for example) may capture a lot of variants, from the high-pitched ones of children to the garbled ones uttered by those with laryngitis. In the speech and hearing sciences, this is called the "magnet effect" of the prototype. Given that its representation is some spatiotemporal pattern in cortex, one can think of this as simply the capture effect of the attractor in the cortical connectivity that produces that characteristic spatiotemporal firing pattern.

Schemas are one kind of fuzzy category. Metaphors are another, and they build upon a foundation of schemas.

Both writers [at the Iowa Writers Workshop] and manics [manic-depressive patients] tend to sort in large

groups, change dimensions while in the process of
sorting, arbitrarily change starting points, or use vague
distantly related concepts as categorizing principles.

NANCY ANDREASEN and PAULINE POWERS, 1975

METAPHORS AND ANALOGICAL REASONING are the central means by
which we project structure across levels. We use schemas as
source domains for constructing a metaphor, as when UP-DOWN is
used in the metaphor MORE IS UP. When we say that the stock
market is up, we refer back to our childhood experiences of
stacking things in a pile, where more things make a higher pile.

When we try to understand one domain of experience in
terms of structures from a different domain, we usually strip some
detail away from the donor. When we metaphorically speak of
the electrons orbiting the atomic nucleus as being like planets
orbiting the sun, we aren't implying that the nucleus is hot and
yellow, only that the geometry bears some resemblance. We're
making use of such schemas as MASSIVE, ATTRACTS, REVOLVES
AROUND, and CIRCLES to help describe something too small to see;
again, structures are more likely to be mapped than mere
attributes.

The power of metaphors, poetic similes, Aesop's parables,
analogies, maps, and economists' models is that they permit us to
carry out reasoning within a familiar domain and subsequently
map our findings back to the domain of interest. The Macintosh
desktop metaphor allowed people to operate in the familiar realm
of folders, documents, and trash cans rather than having to think
about those pesky directories, files, and deletions.

If analogies map with enough points of correspondence, you
can reason with some accuracy. You can solve electrical problems,
for example, using the analogy to water flow [or, if you prefer, the
analogy to moving crowds]. An object such as a *wire* maps to a
pipe [or a sidewalk]. Properties map too: electrical *current* maps
to flow rate [or the rate at which people pass a checkpoint]; *voltage*
maps to water pressure [or to the push of the crowd]; resistance
can be narrow pipes [or sidewalk cafes that obstruct]. Relations
can be imported as well: we can *connect* wires much as we do
pipes [or pathways].

To serve as the source domain of a metaphor, a schema needs to be pervasive in our experience, well understood, and simply structured. Anyone who teaches is constantly on the lookout for useful metaphors, but most candidates have to be discarded because their source domain isn't simply structured or isn't familiar enough. More people can solve electrical circuit problems using the crowd-flow analogy, probably because few of us are sufficiently experienced with fluid dynamics for it to be a good source domain. With such an analogy, you can often guess the answer to parallel resistor and source impedance problems.

Schemas constrain our meaning and understanding. If we take CIRCLE too literally in our quest for understanding orbiting electrons, we will miss out on elliptical paths. Metaphors similarly constrain our reasoning: MORE IS UP might blind us to enormous underground fungi. Mark Johnson's analysis of Hans Selye's work on stress emphasizes how the BODY AS MACHINE metaphor in medicine (breakdowns occur at specific points in the system, repair may involve replacement or mending, etc.) blinded physiologists for a long time because there was no locale for purpose in a machine. Switching to the HOMEOSTASIS metaphor (up-regulating, down-regulating within components) allowed Selye to envisage a widely distributed system associated with response to stress and then predict some of its malfunctions.

But constraints are also the strength of schemas and metaphors, in the sense of a channel, within which the mapping can wander with a loose fit. You can be more-or-less "in the groove." This is reminiscent of basins of attraction, where many starting paths eventually "converge," allowing us to imagine a relatively standard spatiotemporal pattern as the underpinning of a schema.

Again, there would seem to be no problem with encoding a metaphor (even a *gedankenexperiment*) as a hexagonal spatio-temporal pattern, much as in the case of other categories. It would just tend to be recombinations of schema codes, rather than those of the more concrete mental images needed for making a schema code. Linkage would be even more important in implementing the metaphor, converting thought into action, but the unit hexagonal representation would be what competes with alternatives.

Before tackling analogical reasoning, let us note that high level concepts involving relationships need not occupy any more space than low level ones for objects. Just as short words and long words can equally well refer to complex concepts, so they can probably all occupy a single pair of adjacent hexagons in cerebral cortex. It's the linkages that must be followed before getting the action underway which may become more extensive at the more abstract levels.

> The problem is that our states of mind are usually subject to change. The properties of physical things tend to persist when their contexts are changed — but the "significance" of a thought, idea, or partial state of mind depends upon which other thoughts are active at the time and upon what eventually emerges from the conflicts and negotiations among one's agencies. It is an illusion to assume a clear and absolute distinction between "expressing" and "thinking," since expressing is itself an active process that involves simplifying and reconstituting a mental state by detaching it from the more diffuse and variable parts of its context.
>
> MARVIN MINSKY, 1987

THE ANALOGICAL REASONING PROBLEM [*A* is to *B* as *C* is to...?] can now be explored in some mechanistic detail, at least as a *gedanken-experiment*. Let us assume that the choices *D, E, F* are either given or generated (in the manner of the candidates for the ambiguous round object that went whizzing past in chapter 6). What are the steps in arriving at an answer — even an incorrect one — assuming hexagonal cloning competitions?

First of all, there is the relationship problem: what attributes are shared by *A* and *B*? Size, animate-inanimate, movement, color, or perhaps one of those exemplar schemas? Let us say that ATTRACTS and CONTAINMENT are prominent among *AB* associations, that BLUE and BLOCKAGE are among *CD*'s, CONTAINMENT and CIRCLES are among *CE*'s, and that *CF* has no schema associations, only less common ones. On this basis, only the *CE* association CONTAINMENT is shared with those of *AB*.

Although this would seem to require a staged series of hexagonal competitions, remember the lessons of plating rows of infectious material and columns of the different antibiotics in order to find matches in the matrix — and, hopefully, an antibiotic that will attack all the organisms involved. Finding rare higher-dimensional combinations in the "directed evolution" experiments of molecular biology can now be done by matching up fragments of DNA with RNA candidates. All we really need, after *CD*, *CE*, and *CF* territories are each formed up, is for them to override an *AB* territory, with its fading attractors in the short-term memory for ATTRACTS and CONTAINMENT. One then reduces the excitability until only the better resonances remain active; *AB*'s fading CONTAINMENT attractor will help keep *CE* going better than its competitors.

One could match for several shared attractors simultaneously without additional staging, thanks to the short-term memory of *AB* biasing the competition. And one can always use successive layers of staging, as in the sashimi example, each fading with time. That gives some additional possibilities, analogous to generations of back-crossing of hybrids to the parent population.

> I sometimes begin a drawing with no preconceived problem to solve, with only the desire to use pencil on paper and make lines, tones and shapes with no conscious aim; but as my mind takes in what is so produced, a point arrives where some idea becomes conscious and crystallizes, and then control and ordering begins to take place.
>
> HENRY MOORE

SHORTCUTTING HEGEMONY REQUIREMENTS may, of course, be common, especially when we quickly react to something familiar. Indeed, a shortcut could be as subcortical as a reflex; many, surely, live in the basal ganglia. But some shortcuts are likely descended from repeated cortical cloning competitions. Might they still bear hallmarks of a hexagonal origin? Might understanding shortcutting allow us to see how an algorithmic procedure can eventually substitute for a cloning competition?

For coupling of thought to action, there will probably be two spatiotemporal patterns involved, a processed sensory stimulus such as *Apple* and a movement program such as SAY "APPLE". I will again use the butterfly attractor as an easily visualized example of how an association can be formed, as two separate attractors become one strange attractor for *Apple*, SAY "APPLE".

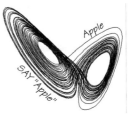

The minimal set of attractors for cloning triangular arrays involves two adjacent hexagons. I will explore the duet case here and rephrase the question: How can a multiple-trial, spatially-extensive, territory of a sensory schema and a movement schema association become, on some future presentation, preemptive? Acting before a substantial territory forms? It depends on how output pathway gating mechanisms interpret "good enough."

Ordinarily, quite a few hexagonal candidates might be reporting at once, with no one set of voices clearly standing out from the crowd in the manner that Brian Eno called "nimble playing." With plenty of time to await a coherent choir to emerge, an economistlike weighing-all-the-factors decision can then be made. But sometimes, you operate very quickly. Consider the rates at which you can comprehend the sentences on this page; surely shortcuts are used for the familiar words, and we only have darwinian competitions when we stumble — and, perhaps, for the highest levels of sentence meaning. Even there, good-enough hegemony may be more like the way committee decisions are informally taken, moving on to some other topic without a formal vote, yet without total agreement of all parties. Only on some occasions is it likely to be like an electoral plurality following a full day of voting.

In the presence of some "hurry up" factor, several strong voices from a small choir, early in the competition period, might suffice for action to be gated in *HurryUp Mode*. How might this be done using a foundation of hexagonal cloning? On the assumption that shortcuts were originally formed via a history of large synchronous choirs, we can ask how that history might modify certain cortical hexagons within a typical territory to make them more successful on their own, during "hurry up" times.

While one characteristic of a successful territory in ordinary competitive times is the size of the recruited choir, no one hexagonal *Apple, SAY "APPLE"* tile of cortex knows how big the entire territory is. But there are core areas, ones that are always activated for *Apple, SAY "APPLE"*, just as there are peripheral patches that are activated on some trials and not others. The core areas are more likely to have complete sets of triangular arrays. And in these core areas, the nodes of triangular arrays might be particularly well-defined, as error correction from crystallization tendencies are presumably at their best there. So these centrally-located hexagons might function particularly well together, seldom impeding neighbors with "off-key" notes.

A perfectly synchronous duet could be easily detected with a sufficiently well-tuned NMDAlike synaptic arrangement in a neuron having a high threshold from an automatic gain control. Although all triangular arrays are approximately synchronous and approximately triangular, the ones repeatedly at the core of a repeatedly large territory might be more sharply defined and truly synchronous — even at startup, before a larger territory forms.

A short but detailed *SAY "APPLE"* melody would probably be needed for a fast track decision. So one can imagine the musical equivalent of a characteristic introductory phrase — say, Beethoven's *dit-dit-dit-dah* — packed into a short period of time. An arpeggio might be a faster *SAY "APPLE"* signature, as it would correspond to a half-dozen pairs of cells all firing in succession rather than the same cells having to fire again, as in the Beethoven example. Fastest of all would be an idiosyncratic chord coming simultaneously from two adjacent hexagons. As such, it would probably be a hash, good for getting the *SAY "APPLE"* movement started but not actually constituting the full movement program; however, details of a movement could follow, after the *Go* decision was made.

Such a preemptive scheme has its dangers. Whenever in *HurryUp Mode*, the organism would be at the mercy of millimeter-sized patches of cerebral cortex, trusting them not to get their act together too quickly, not to pop into the *Apple, SAY "APPLE"* spatio-temporal pattern unless an apple were truly present and the situation appropriate. If *Apple* were even a little ambiguous, you'd want the *Apple, SAY "APPLE"* linkage to be delayed long enough by competitors for other such strange attractors to get there first.

As such, it becomes a reaction time problem, where it is very desirable to have short latencies for sure bets and longer latencies for the others. Longer latencies, in the hexagonal theory, result from having to clone more territory before synchrony, from crystallization tendencies that sharpen things up, and from linkage requirements.

A COMMON NEURAL MACHINERY, for many tasks involving fancy structured sequences, is something that I have discussed elsewhere. Most of the ballistic limb movements (not flinging, but the more accurate forms of hammering, clubbing, kicking, and especially throwing) need extensive planning because, as noted earlier, the feedback loop takes so long that the motion is about finished before the initial feedback starts to correct the movement. Certainly correcting the timing of the higher velocity parts of such movements is a task for a subsequent performance, not the current one. One way to reduce the performance variability is to use a lot of clones of the right movement command, halving the jitter with every quadrupling of the chorus size.

If evolution provides you with the neural machinery for doing one such task, maybe it can be used at other times for constructing the structures needed for language and planning ahead. Ape-to-human evolution during the last six million years may well have involved natural selection "for" all these skills at various times. A common neural substrate has an interesting implication. Improving one skill via enlargement might also improve the others, for example, selection for language skills could improve throwing accuracy (and vice versa, which I consider even more likely). Some uses of this common neural machinery for fancy structured sequences, such as music and dance and games, have probably been under little environmental selection for their own usefulness.

Hexagonal cloning competitions seem possible for many cortical areas; they all, so far, have some version of the spatially patterned intrinsic horizontal connections in the superficial layers that, together with entrainment tendencies, provide the setup for synchronized triangular arrays. Language localization in cortex is highly variable among individuals, suggesting a widespread substrate of cortical areas that are capable of housing the particular attractors that form up to implement language during the preschool years. So too, planning and the ballistic skills might have a variable localization — and be able to borrow nonspecialist areas on occasion.

LAYERS OF MIDDLEMEN are familiar from everyday economics, and we expect to see many layers of representation standing between our consciousness and the real world. As Derek Bickerton noted:

> [T]he more consciousness one has, the more layers of
> processing divide one from the world. . . . Progressive
> distancing from the external world is simply the price that is
> paid for knowing anything about the world at all. The deeper
> and broader [our] consciousness of the world becomes, the
> more complex the layers of processing necessary to obtain that
> consciousness.

But we are also increasingly familiar with the tendency toward disintermediation (producers or wholesale warehouses selling directly to the public).

The useful mental shortcut is also disintermediation. Sometimes it conflates several different levels of explanation (the results of mingling the levels can be either good or bad). Even more important than shortcuts may be consolidation, creating a firm footing which allows the exploration of new complexities. This Rube Goldberg tower of the quasi-stable is what Jacob Bronowski liked to call stratified stability.

Stage-setting and warm-up exercises are probably an important preamble to operating in the metaphorical realm. With particularly good metaphorical stand-ins for the real world, we can even simulate courses of action before coming to closure, acting for real. A decision is usually a "good enough" judgment but it varies with the setting, *Bingo* on some perfect-fit occasions and "Let's get on with it" when comparisons have exhausted themselves.

KNOWING THAT THE TEMPERATURE OUTSIDE is 26 °C may not do you much good, unless you compare it to room temperature, or to your own criterion for short-sleeve-shirt temperature. "Compared to what" can also save you from impulsive decisions, such as selecting a box of breakfast cereal that costs twice as much per serving as beefsteak. A politician's statement may sound fine, until you compare it to what was said to other people or in earlier times. The James Thurber aphorism, "You can fool too many of the people too much of the time," is all about a common lack of "Compared to what?" — and how others exploit it for votes or profit.

Half of education seems, at times, to consist of cultivating a habit of mind that avoids premature closure — to do some comparison shopping, at least for long enough to involve some standard schemas such as BEFORE-AFTER. When selecting a rental car at the airport counter, we invoke LARGER-SMALLER and so bring to mind some comfort considerations — and also the memory that many garages now have undersized parking spaces, meaning that small cars will fit into all of the empty spaces while the large car will need to pass up half of the candidates.

Then the MORE-LESS schema brings up rental costs, and BETTER-WORSE reminds us of considerations such as crash worthiness and poor design. Because there are a limited number of schemas, invoking them may eventually become "hardwired" in a way that fancier comparisons cannot. Indeed, schemas might not even require hexagonal cloning competitions, because they have become so routinized that ordinary weighing criteria suffice (and so, because the clock is ticking away, we pick the intermediate-sized rental car, once again).

It's meeting a high quality criteria that, in the end, makes a judgment emotionally satisfying, whether it is detecting complicated patterns or creating fancy maneuvers. In some areas, quality

is judged against elaborate criteria, not just routine schemas.
Whatever rationality consists of, its classy reputation is surely tied
up with narrative structure, with our quest for narrative unity,
and how well we satisfy it.

We are evidently unique among species in our symbolic ability,
and we are certainly unique in our modest ability to control the
conditions of our existence by using these symbols. Our ability
to represent and simulate reality implies that we can
approximate the order of existence and bring it to serve human
purposes. A good simulation, be it a religious myth or
scientific theory, gives us a sense of mastery over our
experience. To represent something symbolically, as we do
when we speak or write, is somehow to capture it, thus making
it one's own. But with this approximation comes the
realization that we have denied the immediacy of reality and
that in creating a substitute we have but spun another thread in
the web of our grand illusion.

HEINZ PAGELS, 1988

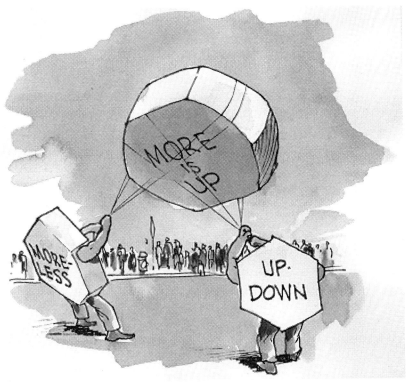

"Ground that metaphor!"

11

Thinking a Thought in the Mosaics of the Mind

We, unlike the cells that compose us, are not on
ballistic trajectories; we are *guided* missiles, capable of
altering course at any point, abandoning goals,
switching allegiances, forming cabals and then
betraying them, and so forth. For us, it is always
decision time, and because we live in a world of memes,
no consideration is alien to us, or a foregone
conclusion.

DANIEL C. DENNETT, 1995

ONCE THEY FINISH WITH THINGS AS BASIC as perceptual transformations and memory phenomena, theories of brain
function must explain abstractions and associations as
diverse as categories, abstracts, schemas, scripts, syntax, and
metaphor. But these too are only intermediate goals for a theory
of higher intellectual function. Any one worthy of the name also
aspires, however sketchily, to explaining the unity of conscious
experience and how it shifts (indeed, can be steered) among topics
that had, shortly before, been gestating subconsciously.

Consciousness, as I have discussed in both *The Cerebral
Symphony* and *How Brains Think*, has so many different common
connotations that discussions are often confusing, everyone
talking at cross purposes. Even within medicine and neuroscience, the word means quite a few different things, and there is
no reason to assume that they share common mechanisms.

Many follow the long neurological tradition of defining
consciousness quite narrowly, as mere awareness, but I think that

we now have the conceptual tools to do better, to approach Piaget's problem of what you use when you don't know what to do. In the Karl Popper formulation of consciousness:

> Much of our purposeful behaviour (and presumably of the purposeful behaviour of animals) happens without the intervention of consciousness. . . . Problems that can be solved by routine do not need consciousness. [The biological achievements that are helped by consciousness are the solution of *problems of a non-routine kind.*] But the role of consciousness is perhaps clearest where an aim or purpose. . . can be achieved by *alternate means,* and when two or more means are tried out, after deliberation.

We are unaware of most of the things that go on in our heads, and sometimes that's better, as in Zen archery. When we really learn a new movement sequence, it seems to become a subroutine that no longer requires conscious attention: tying a necktie or hair ribbon required lots of conscious attention in the beginning, but once established (perhaps at a subcortical level) we can do it better if we don't try to think about it. What is, initially, consciously mediated can become subconscious with practice.

But our subconscious tasks run a spectrum from the expert to the amateur, even the random. Here we need to address both the expert subroutine that no longer requires conscious attention and the subconscious candidates that are being shaped up for quality — one of which eventually succeeds in replacing the current content of consciousness as it fades.

A *gedankenexperiment* for consciousness in this broader sense is where this final chapter is heading, but let us first examine the security of the footing that this darwinian patchwork quilt has provided for such a necessarily ambitious extrapolation.

> LONG before the reader has arrived at this part of my work, a crowd of difficulties will have occurred to him. Some of them are so serious that to this day I can hardly reflect on them without being in some degree staggered; but, to the best of my judgment, the greater number are only apparent, and those that are real are not, I think, fatal to the theory.
>
> CHARLES DARWIN, 1859

THE FIRST TASK OF ANY THEORY is to economically account for the descriptions, to cover a certain group of facts. The extent of coverage of a theory is easily overestimated when the foundations are not specifiable. Some theories are reminiscent of fortune cookie wisdom: surely true at some place, at some time, in some sense. The lack of specification of the when-where-why details makes fortunes not terribly useful. We need details to avoid the theoretical trap of premature closure, which leaves us holding a fortune-cookie explanation that specifies little.

For a brain theory, economical description is a particularly demanding task because of the need to span multiple levels of mechanism — from synapses to cells to circuits to modules, and more. And also span multiple levels of phenomenological explanation — such as attributes, objects, categories, analogies, and metaphors.

Beyond this descriptive aspect, a theory tries to predict, whenever possible, features not yet observed. Prediction is a minor aspect of historical theories such as evolutionary theory, but it is always valued as a shortcut, its failures warning that it is perhaps time to try another formulation. Yet biology is full of exceptions to rules, and so theoretical predictions are more likely to be valued for the experimental strategies they suggest than they are for strategic tests in the falsification mode.

A number of predictions have fallen out of neocortical hexagons, suggesting various experimental handles. If the reader will indulge me in another celebratory recapitulation, I'll run through a selection of the theory's predictions, together with some related descriptive successes.

AS A DESCRIPTIVE THEORY, neocortical hexagons can explicitly account for Hebb's dual trace memory, with characteristic spatio-temporal patterns for immediate memory and attractors embedded in the synaptic connectivity for the memories lasting minutes and lifetimes. It also describes one aspect of the widely distributed synchrony that has been observed in cortex. As a predictive theory, it offers synchronized triangular arrays extending their reach as the key prediction amenable to present recording techniques.

The hexagons theory describes why many short-term memories might not be successfully stored as long-term memories. It is consistent with the senile dementias that seemingly uncover long-ago memories during a period when no new short-term memories are being created. It predicts strategies for enhancing storage and recall, as in the sashimi staging of fading attractors.

It describes redundancy of memory sites, describes the slow loss or modification of memories with age via the redundancy being reduced by overlain attractors. It predicts slowed access times when fewer pairs of adjacent hexagons remain that possess the same attractor within their repertoire.

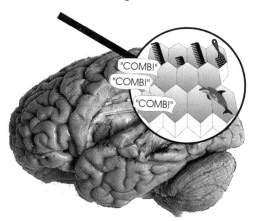

It describes simple associations of sensory schemas with movement program schemas. It predicts that this association could occur in convergence zones via superposition of active firing patterns, or melding of attractors — but, thanks to the *faux* fax, the linkage could even happen in sensory or motor cortices.

It describes one aspect of cortical plasticity following stroke, via multifunctionality coexisting with specialization of cortical areas. It predicts that an expert region could, by simply altering the slant of the triangular arrays, avoid the local permanent connectivity specialties — and thereby function temporarily as a more general purpose work space. It predicts that a given cortical area could have multiple "personalities" corresponding to different slants of the triangular arrays.

It describes some of the functional roles associated with mini-columns and macrocolumns. It predicts a new type of macro-column-sized, hexagonal-shaped functional structure in association cortex that, unlike other macrocolumns, may overlap with one another.

It describes the general features of the spontaneous activity seen with microelectrode techniques in association cortex: usually random in timing and low in average firing rate, with silence the norm. It predicts that sources centimeters apart in a given cortical area could, via interdigitating triangular arrays, create unit spatio-temporal patterns about 0.5 mm across, ones that repeat as in wallpaper. It predicts that the attractor circuitry critical for the re-creation of the spatiotemporal patterns in recall can be compacted from map-sized circuitry into macrocolumnar-sized structures, with much redundancy also achieved.

It describes why recurrent excitation among superficial pyram-idal neurons should be associated with NMDA synapses, LTP, and standard distance gaps in the intrinsic horizontal connections. It suggests automatic gain controls that prevent runaway recruit-ment and, more uniquely, it predicts that the nodes of triangular arrays should shrink over time. It predicts that central regions should crystallize into closer approximations to equilateral triangles (remembering, of course, the "good-enough" caution, p. 36) as territories enlarge.

It describes retrograde inhibition of memories, where a new telephone number may impede your access to the old one, via chaotic capture. It predicts that regional reductions in excitability could erase immediate memories, while leaving fading basins of attraction from which active patterns could be rekindled.

It describes how seizures could fog recent memories, in the manner of road resurfacing filling in the gaps in the road that constitute the washboard pattern, or in the manner that edema can obscure characteristic facial wrinkles. It predicts that maintaining a widespread nonsensical "mantra" pattern for the duration of neocortical LTP could, by minimizing meaningful associations, serve to prevent other temporary attractors from forming.

It describes both *déjà vu* and premature closure; it predicts that an agnosia could be created by a similar clone-too-quickly mechanism that preempts slower links from affecting the outcome.

It describes the long reaction times (so improbable merely from conduction delays) of cognitive processing via the time it takes for synchronization, local recruitment, and cross-modality links via convergence zones. It predicts a shortening of such times via cross-modality priming.

It describes neural equivalents of simple mutations and deletions (the "capacity to blunder slightly") and predicts some equivalents of recombination via active superpositions by triangular array interdigitation. It predicts passive superpositions via successively-overlain attractors. It predicts geometrical arrangements of barriers and battle fronts whereby otherwise sterile hybrids might reproduce themselves.

It describes the construction and deconstruction of attributes, objects, schemas, and even analogies; like Hebb's cell-assembly theory applied to stabilized image fragmentation, it has features of both the holistic and specialization views of mental function. It predicts multiple levels of stratified stability, each able to use darwinian processes to improve quality and create novelties, some of which could constitute a heightened form of consciousness.

THE DIFFERENT LEVELS OF EXPLANATION and mechanism are important to distinguish, if we are to avoid the confusions of level (and all the arguing at cross purposes) that marked evolutionary biology in the several decades after the rediscovery of Mendel's genetics in 1900. Eventually most came to see mutations and selectionism as two sides of the same coin rather than competing explanations, but it took a few decades. As Jonathan Weiner wrote in *The Beak of the Finch*:

> After Darwin's death, many biologists found it easy to accept evolution and impossible to accept Darwin's chief explanation for it. Evolution, yes; selection, no. William Bateson, the founder of modern genetics, wrote an elegy for Darwinism in 1913, calling it "so inapplicable to the facts that we can only marvel. . . at the want of penetration displayed by the advocates of such a proposition."

This was one of the inspirations for J. B. S. Haldane's wonderful quip about "the four stages of acceptance of a scientific theory: (i) this is worthless nonsense; (ii) this is an interesting, but perverse, point of view; (iii) this is true, but quite unimportant; (iv) I always said so." These days, confusing variation with selection is on a par with confusing genotype and phenotype, something that biologists (but few others) successfully avoid.

It took three decades before the Neodarwinian Evolutionary Synthesis straightened out our thinking about the relationship between genetics and darwinism, between individuals and populations; hopefully we won't have to go though it again when talking about milliseconds-to-minutes darwinism. However, ignorance about levels of explanation abounds, particularly in recent writings about quantum mechanics as a basis for consciousness, showing how attractive these confusions of level can be. In *How Brains Think*, I call the most grandiose confusion "the Janitor's Dream." (Hoping to leap from the subbasement of quantum mechanics to the penthouse of consciousness in a single bound!)

For milliseconds-to-minutes darwinism, the most reasonable confusion is surely with the days-to-years selectionism that Changeux and Edelman describe so well for wiring up the nervous system in ontogeny, and for selecting useful modifications of that wiring by lifetime experience. I have tended to describe this level as involving modifications of the attractors; other terms associated with these long-term spatial-only patterns are bumps and ruts in the washboarded road, synaptic weights, and connectionism.

Differential alterations of synaptic strengths are surely happening much as described, and Edelman's reentrant interactions with "cortical appendendages" are likely a major mechanism for editing and emphasis, much in the manner of the sculpturing selectionism of William James a century earlier:

The mind is at every stage a theatre of simultaneous possibilities. Consciousness consists in the comparison of these with each other, the selection of some, and the suppression of the rest by the reinforcing and inhibiting agency of attention. The highest and most elaborated mental products are filtered from the data chosen by the faculty next beneath, out of the mass offered by the faculty below that, which mass in turn was sifted from a still larger amount of yet simpler material, and so on. The mind, in short, works on the data it receives very much as a sculptor works on his block of stone.

Note that mine is not a rival theory to such forms of neural selectionism (except insofar as they claim to extend to the James-Piaget-Popper aspect of consciousness). Rather, the ephemeral copying competitions that I emphasize rest on the broad foundation of such longer-term selectionism, which forms part of the environment that biases cloning success (and *faux* faxing) on my short time scale of milliseconds to minutes. As such, my ephemeral copying competitions are one layer up from the connectionist layer, though they feed back to it when altering the synaptic strengths, just as Edelman's reentry also shapes connectivity changes.

HEGEMONY IS WHAT ESTABLISHES THE TOPIC of our current conscious experience, in the present theory; the remaining mosaics of other patterns constitute our subconscious. Leadership or dominance, especially of one state over another, seems applicable to cortical territories as well as to nation-states. Eventually, if no sensory input demands attention, one of the nondominant patterns will take over from the current winner, perhaps a pattern that is novel, with no basis in existing memories, perhaps one that represents a familiar worry.

E PLURIBUS UNUM
"Out of many, one"
(Latin motto of the USA)

Passive awareness (and its neural correlates) may be much simpler than the creative constructs implied by the James-Piaget-Popper levels of consciousness; a pop-through recognition of a familiar object may not need to utilize a cloning competition in the manner of an ambiguous percept or a novel movement. Hexagonal mosaics surely aren't everything going on in the brain; indeed, they are probably just one mode of operation of some expanses of neocortex, and regulated by other brain regions such as hippocampus and thalamus. But here-this-minute, gone-the-next mosaics seem quite suitable for explaining many aspects of mind, aspects that have been difficult to imagine emerging from quantum mechanics, chemistry, neurotransmitters, single neurons, simple circuits, or even the smaller neocortical modules such as minicolumns. In some regions, at some times, hexagonal competitions might be the main thing happening. They're a level of explanation that looks as if it might be appropriate; we'll have to see just how far we can go with it as an explanation for talking-to-yourself consciousness.

Edelman quite reasonably forswears a treatment of thought itself at one point (this may seem surprising in a book claiming to be about consciousness, but remember those self-imposed blinders of the neurological tradition). He proceeds to define thought as the building of conceptual theories about the world. I too would emphasize process over product, though I would also include those events at the lower end of the quality scale — the process during the four hours of mulling-things-over each night (half of all sleep) that rarely makes any progress and that of the fantastic juxtapositions of our episodes of dreaming sleep. At the high end, I would emphasize the progressive shaping up of quality, the discovery of order among seeming disorder, and the creation of new levels of abstraction for relationships.

With hexagonal copying competitions, one can sketch out what the thought process might involve, using neocortical aspects of (1) spatio-temporal patterns of active firing and (2) the attractors embedded in the connectivity (thought will, of course, also involve the thalamocortical loops

The proper, unique, and perpetual object of thought: that which does not exist, that which is not before me, that which was, that which will be, that which is possible, that which is impossible.
PAUL VALÉRY

and those cortical appendages, what I have perhaps too briefly subsumed under extrinsic biases to the basins of attraction). Thought might not be very different in principle from what I sketched out in the ambiguous object example of classification (p. 90), with its problem of finding candidates and then making a decision among them. Just imagine ideas competing for space, rather than the cerebral codes for candidate objects.

A major difference, however, is that thought may have to span many levels of explanation and locate an appropriate one. As we try to speak usefully about a subject, we are often torn between dwelling on rock-solid details and speaking in perhaps-too-abstract generalities. In a book-length work, one may range over the spectrum — though readers may not always synchronously co-vary in their preferences for details and overviews!

THEORIES ABOUT THE MIND not only have to explain capabilities; they also have to be consistent with what we know about pathological processes. This book is not the place for an extended discourse on those features of neurological and psychiatric illnesses that might involve cloning competitions. Among the things that could go wrong are the speed of cloning, the rate of interruptions, the magnitude of such climate changes, the plurality needed for a winner, the duration of the ephemeral mosaic, the duration of fading short-term attractors, the local ratios of neuromodulators, and all of the same things via the inherently noisy *faux* fax linkages. A few examples may serve to indicate the handles available for experimental design.

> Men ought to know that from nothing else but the brain come joys, delights, laughter and sports, and sorrows, griefs, despondency, and lamentations.... And by the same organ we become mad.
>
> HIPPOCRATES

> To study the abnormal is the best way of understanding the normal.
>
> WILLIAM JAMES

Although the "Janitor's Dream" may be improbable, some leaping between nonadjacent levels is surely allowed within the neocortical representation levels, just from the nature of cerebral codes in the hexagonal theory. There's really nothing to keep the cerebral code for *Apple* from competing with that of *Fruit*. We all make categorical mistakes, then try to weed them out. One simple pathology would be the failure to weed before speaking, as in the illogicality and non sequiturs of positive formal thought disorder.

Should the neocortex be too excitable, few barriers to cloning will form. That means even fewer gateways; not as many variants will escape error correction, and so the solution space will be only briefly explored. You'd be able to colonize large areas without competition along the way. Besides making for results of poor quality, the spatiotemporal pattern that succeeds may have the large homogenous "choir" normally associated with successful memory recalls. Even situations that were unfamiliar might thereby seem familiar. *Déjà vu* experiences might be one result.

Should the cortex be insufficiently excitable, routine tasks might still operate but tasks that required concentration or sorting through possibilities would be greatly slowed. Few new episodic memories would form, and amnesia might be a typical complaint.

Patchy versions of too little or too much might give rise to dissociations and fugue states. The patient who finds himself in San Francisco, but is unable to remember why he traveled there, may have a substantial roadblock (an extensive barrier region, without U-paths available) in his cortex, or have dead end detours (attractor basins that divert attempts to approach those memories).

Infrequent changes have an interesting pathology as well, even when average amounts are normal. Inability to form a large choir, as might occur when excitability fluctuations are minimized and allow stalemates to persist, would give rise to other types of thought pathology, such as indecision and inappropriate unfamiliarity judgments (suggesting *jamais vu*). If "climate changes" are an important part of the rapidity of recognition or decision making, some subcortical pathologies might have their effects on cortex by insufficient fluctuations, rather than from insufficient average levels of cortical input. Or their fluctuations might be too slow.

Too frequent changes, of course, suggest accelerated variation and decision making — and bring to mind a classic form of mental disorder, the rapidity of thought associated with manic-depressive illness.

> There is a particular kind of pain, elation, loneliness, and terror involved in this kind of madness. When you're high it's tremendous. The ideas and feelings are fast and frequent like shooting stars, and you follow them until you find better and brighter ones. Shyness goes, the right words and gestures are suddenly there, the power to captivate others a felt certainty. There are interests found in uninteresting people. Sensuality is

pervasive and the desire to seduce and be seduced irresistible. Feelings of ease, intensity, power, well-being, financial omnipotence, and euphoria pervade one's marrow. But, somewhere, this changes. The fast ideas are far too fast, and there are far too many; overwhelming confusion replaces clarity. Memory goes. Humor and absorption on friends' faces are replaced by fear and concern. Everything previously moving with the grain is now against - you are irritable, angry, frightened, uncontrollable, and enmeshed totally in the blackest caves of the mind. You never knew those caves were there.

KAY REDFIELD JAMISON, 1995

RAPIDITY OF THOUGHT, in most of us, varies a great deal. The phrase, however, has a special meaning in psychiatry. An expert (someone that knows all the common mistakes and how to avoid them) may be able to operate quickly in a way that the amateur cannot. But the speed variations in someone with manic-depressive illness (or its less extreme relative, cyclothymia) may have nothing to do with how well established the links are. Even an expert, dealing with familiar material, may go from a fluidity of making connections and decisions in hypomania to a slow, labored train of thought in depression, lingering too long and failing to make obvious connections with what is obviously there (as too-late recall eventually proves).

The effectiveness of the antidepressant medications suggests, of course, that depressed mood might involve imbalances in the major neuromodulators, especially the norepinephrine and sero-tonin systems. But the existence of mixed depression keeps us from making a simple equation of retarded thought with mood: in many bipolar and cyclothymic patients, racing thoughts and pressured speech can occur in both high and low states. In hypomania, every new idea may seem promising; in mixed depression, equally frequent thoughts may be systematically devalued and so one quickly thinks one's way into a gloomy cave.

While the cortical hexagons theory has nothing to say, at present, about global influences on mood or alertness in the manner of Hobson's theory, it does offer a number of candidates for rapidity of thought (all of those analogs to climate change and island biogeography) and making connections (via the *faux* fax mechanism and those $N_k < N_a$ linkage requirements). One can easily imagine additional ones, equivalents of boredom or novelty-seeking, that might be associated with the number of simultaneous contenders or the "generation time."

> The experimental subjects in isolation saw, among other things, primitive animals in a prehistoric jungle and modern squirrels wearing snowshoes. . . . Charles Lindbergh in his solitary flight across the Atlantic was aware of "ghostly presences riding in my airplane" and "vapor-like shapes crowding the fuselage, speaking with human voices, giving me advice and important messages." Solitary sailors, and survivors of shipwreck in lifeboats, report having visions. Even on land, in apparently normal circumstances, the monotony of long-distance car-driving on the Western plains of the North American continent may lead the driver to see things — jackrabbits big enough to step over the car in one case — and the long-distance truck-driver at night following that endless white line down the highway may wreck his truck trying to avoid collision with a nonexistent object on the highway before him.
>
> DONALD O. HEBB, 1980

THOUGHT DISORDERS involve psychosis without a concomitant mood change. The two hallmarks of psychosis are hallucinations (not counting those of obvious cause, such as Lindbergh's) and delusions. Hallucinations are where imagined events or memory recalls come to be mistaken for current sensory input: voices may be heard, burning sensations felt, shapes or people seen. Enthusiasts have been known to seek them out via dehydration, sweat baths, drugs, and sensory deprivation.

Tuberculosis used to be a major hallucinogenic disease, via tuberculomas of the temporal lobe; the voices that Joan of Arc heard were likely due to this. Today, schizophrenia, manic-depressive illness, and epilepsy are the brain disorders producing most of the unprompted hallucinations (though we all, of course, experience psychotic symptoms with every REM-episode dream). To understand a mechanistic foundation for thought is, hopefully, to pave the way to appreciating and modifying the intrusive thoughts of schizophrenia. The hexagonal cloning theory suggests that the content of a hallucination is only the stuff of subconscious contention, that the pathology might consist of it being taken seriously, premature closure occurring before quality can be shaped up.

Delusions are more subtle, long-term failures of reality testing than are hallucinations. The common delusions are of persecution, jealousy, grandiosity, sin and guilt — like hallucinations in dreams, we all experience them; the pathology is more a matter of persistence. In schizophrenia, they can extend to bizarre notions that have no basis in anyone's experience, such as being controlled by men from Mars. And why is the delusion not overwritten by corrections, all those things that usually modify our erroneous judgments with further experience? Or discounted, as we regularly ignore our nighttime dreams? Why doesn't an *idée fixe* fade, like my unused calculus theorems? A delusion often seems as intransigent as any innate tendency with which we are born, difficult to ignore or unlearn.

The delusion (or, for that matter, the obsession or compulsion) could be from a particularly secure basin of attraction. A particularly broad catchment, so that many situations are distorted to fit the mold, their cerebral codes captured and standardized in the way that a black hole captures neighbors and renders them invisible, would result in delusionlike properties. Might a delusion's setup involve unusually widespread clones of the attractor, many hundreds scattered over the connectivity of an entire Area, perhaps from some long-ago success that created a large choir that practiced too regularly? From particularly frequent recall, that served to embed the memory even more thoroughly, or obscured approach routes to other basins of attraction?

THE META-THEORY FOR HEXAGONAL CLONING COMPETITIONS is, at present, like talking about the weather. Subcortical supervisors for quilting seem likely, but some neocortical regions might also tend to supervise the cloning competitions of others, regulate their habituation, and so forth.

Yet it need not be some grand supervisor with even more intelligence. Until something fancier is clearly indicated, the default assumption ought to be that any regulatory process is essentially stupid, perhaps only chaotic phenomena on a grander or slower scale. As they say in many locales, "If you don't like the weather, just wait an hour." The marked seasons of the temperate zones have probably been important in species evolution and we may yet come to say, "If you don't like the climate, just wait a decade." As I argue in *How Brains Think,* the abrupt climate changes superimposed on the ice ages may have helped conserve an inefficient ape variant that happened to be a jack-of-all-trades, able to adapt to new diets within a generation. In cortex, changing the name of the game could happen on the milliseconds-to-minutes time scale.

As such, the electroencephalogram may serve as a useful indicator. We are accustomed to eschewing any functional assignment to the various EEG rhythms, but hexagonal cloning may allow us to view the EEG in a new light — as drivers of territorial expansion and deme extinction.

IF SO MANY THINGS are happening at once in the neocortex, why do we have a unity of conscious experience? We speak with a single voice, even if only talking to ourselves. We have a sense of being at the center of a convergence of various narratives that we use to explain the past, all while trying to choose between several speculative scenarios about the future.

There are some trivial answers to the unity question — as when we say that some things, such as sensing one's blood pressure, are totally inaccessible to verbal reporting mechanisms — and so perhaps the unity is an illusion, simply a problem with what's accessible to verbal report.

In the context of cloning competitions, a more tempting answer is to say that we have a unity of consciousness because there can be only one winner of a competition — and that it's simply the largest patch of the dozens currently to be found somewhere on the dynamically reforming patchwork quilt (or, at least, it's the largest one with ready access to output pathways). If stalemates are prevented by perturbations from the fickle climate, there's always a winner and it's only a question of your threshold for converting thought into action, your quality criterion. So the center of consciousness shifts about, from one cortical area to others, as the train of thought

The imagination is the weather of the mind.
WALLACE STEVENS, 1957

progresses. This neatly explains why no neocortical lesion seems able to abolish consciousness, only to abolish certain types of content such as color attributes.

But if one phrases the consciousness question as a competition, then of course one gets a unitary answer. Perhaps we should re-phrase the question: Can we possibly do two consciousness-level tasks at the same time? With a theory like spatially distributed cloning competitions, the answer is surely, "Why not?"

That's because the theory suggests various shaping-up competitions proceeding in parallel. If you can have simultaneous quarter-finals and semi-finals leading up to a brain-wide championship that we call the current content of consciousness, then why not simply simultaneously output both the global winner and the second-best from some other area, operating on a different train of thought?

WE WOULD NOT BE EASILY PERSUADED that someone had a "two-track consciousness" if he merely claimed that he could attend to two vigilance tasks simultaneously. Or keep two schemas in mind, one visual and one verbal. We'd require sentence-like tasks. Two simultaneous narratives would be the most persuasive. If consciousness involves generating novelty and selecting between alternative courses of action (rather than consciousness as mere awareness), the demonstration would need two such tasks proceeding in parallel.

But comprehension tasks are usually easier than production tasks: most of us can read a book while listening to the radio. What we need are two simultaneous production-task *outputs* from consciousness-demanding processes. Imagine, for example, a sign language interpreter who, when not interpreting spoken language into sign language, finds it possible to carry on two conversations at the same time, speaking to one person and signing to another. Or a touch typist conducting an internet dialogue with someone on another continent, while talking about something else with a person in the same room.

It wouldn't be interesting if the phenomenon turned out to merely be a matter of clever time-sharing, or of rote replays of memorized material. But, were we able to rule out such less-interesting explanations, a two-track success would suggest an interesting interpretation: that our seeming unity of conscious-ness is simply a matter of most of us having only one major output track available for unique representations (such as reporting on our current thoughts) — and that said pathway has a serial-order bottleneck that admits of only one completed thought at a time.

Not having two independent output paths means that most of us get little experience in managing two trains of thought simult-aneously; we can only use "on the other hand" tactics. But if we became experienced in managing two semi-independent tracks, thanks to several output paths to feed, then two internal voices might also be able to converse with one another.

THOUGH INDEPENDENT SIMULTANEOUS OUTPUTS may be infrequent, simultaneous competitions that influence one another are prob-ably common. We regularly evolve our sentences into "good stories" at the paragraph or page level, applying the quality criteria associated with narrative and epic to guide our product-ions toward satisfying endings. (I'm doing that right here — and certainly in the forthcoming finale.) Why not also evolve them to meet some nonstandard criteria that itself evolves, on a somewhat slower time scale? Using a darwinian copying competition with short-term memories that fade much more slowly?

Indeed, there are some situations that might qualify for such two-level interactive evolution, such as the orbital frontal cortex role in monitoring progress on an agenda, a meta-sequence that seems to tick along on a different time scale than individual thoughts and sentences. There's no requirement that darwinian variations have to be random; a slow darwinian process could bias the general direction of the variants of a faster darwinian process. There could be a cascade or web of such darwinian processes.

THINKING A THOUGHT, in this theory, is more than just a current competition between the cerebral codes that have cloned mosaic territories. It involves the recent history of such competitions, plating the various work spaces with attractors that then fade. It involves biases from moods and from agendas evolving elsewhere. And it involves the attractors of long-term memories, different in different areas.

Habituation processes in dominant areas may allow second-best areas to take over a moment later. Just as neuromodulators serve to sculpt one motor circuit from a network with many possible motor circuits, and so set up an action, the faster-acting synaptic modifications may also help move our attention from a present topic to a new one, from one second to the next.

From the sashimi layering of fading attractors, we may get the appearance of a single-minded person inside, steering the train of thought and stage managing our purposeful behavior. Our current mental state is always unique because, even if we are thinking exactly the same thought as we did yesterday, those fading patterns underlying its spatiotemporal patterns differ in strength and spatial distribution from that of yesterday's sashimi. They will lead the train of thought somewhere else.

While I think that a Darwin Machine operates in the brain and can account for much of higher intellectual function, I am not equally certain that making frequent use of the darwinian algorithm is what elevated us from the ape level of mental abilities — or, for that matter, that it alone is what allows us to operate quickly enough to escape *esprit de l'escalier*. It may be that some shortcuts, cortical or subcortical, are absolutely essential in order for the darwinian process to operate quickly enough to produce useful results within the time span of short-term memory. Those shortcuts might structure agendas and the ascending levels of abstraction, or keep us from constantly backsliding into a hopeless muddle. I suspect that much of fleshing out this theory will involve the theoretical, experimental, and neurological identification of shortcuts, that much of its application to education will involve learning how to augment or avoid them.

An example of a shortcut would be that set of constraints on word order known as syntax. I'm not thinking of plural and past tense formation so much as phrase structure. There's a lot of embedding of phrases, as in a sentence such as *What you see is what you get*, where both the subject and the object are themselves sentences. Embedding is a key step up in beyond-the-apes language abilities.

PROTOLANGUAGE IS A SIMPLE FORM of language lacking the structure provided by syntax. It's the language of the trained apes, children less than two years of age, speakers of pidgins, Broca's aphasics, and American professors trying to communicate with Greek shopkeepers. The difference isn't just vocabulary. With structureless protolanguage, it takes a lot of time to relate who did what to whom, even when supplemented by gestures.

The linguist Derek Bickerton suggests that there are no real intermediates between protolanguage and our full-fledged syntactic language. This raises the issue of what improved neural mechanism could make such a large difference — and I have one to suggest. This isn't the place for serious linguistics or paleo-anthropology, but, given eleven chapters of hexagons to warm up the reader, it is possible to develop a mechanistic outline for much of Universal Grammar (features common to all known languages except pidgins) in just a few more pages.

A NOUN AND ITS MODIFIERS, such as *black shoe*, could be implement-ed by simple borderline superpositions of hexagons. Superimpose this modified noun upon the code for *with* and you have a prepos-itional phrase. Keep going and you might achieve a territory of clones, each of which represents *the tall blond man with one black shoe*. By this point, however, you are well out of the range for do-ing all the association via superpositions at a borderline between territories; that would merely pour all of the words into a blender and leave only a general impression of the intended topic, one that becomes even less specific as more associations are added.

The *faux* fax would seem, at first glimpse, to produce an even more ambiguous superposition. But bi-directional corticocortical links allow you to have your cake and eat it too. Back projections (six out of seven neocortical areas are reciprocally linked) can use the same code, and so immediately contribute to maintaining a chorus above a critical size (they are, presumably, always adapting and thereby falling silent).

It would be like missing choir practice but participating via a conference phone call. The central chorus of *What you see is what you get* could have two subsidiary choruses for *see* and *get*, each implementing appropriate roles for its verb; if either subchorus falters, the top-level one stumbles.

A backprojected spatiotemporal pattern might not need to be fully featured, nor fully synchronized, to help out with the peripheral site's chorus. It could be more like that sing-along technique where a single voice prompts the next verse in a monotone and the chorus repeats it with melodic elaboration; some singing at a fifth or an octave above the others, some with a delay, and so forth. The backpath could include more code than the subchorus uses, just as choirmasters and folk singers manage to include exhortations with the desired text.

Back projections provide a way of resolving any ambiguity associated with recursive embedding by maintaining an audit trail. ("Who mentioned *X*? Sing it again, the whole thing!") With such structuring, there's no longer a danger that the mental model of the eight-word amalgamation *the tall blond man with one black shoe* will be scrambled into a blond black man with one tall shoe.

LINKS CAN ALSO IMPLEMENT THE BINDING needed for words such as *he*, *himself*, and *each other*, whose referents may be in preceding sentences. That's another of the linguists' desiderata, along with a neural mechanism for the *Wh*-question's long-range dependencies. But at the very top of their Universal Grammar wish list is recursive embedding, needed to nest one sentence inside another. (*I think I saw him leave to go home.*)

What keeps the top-level *think* verb's hexagon happy enough to reproduce effectively in a copying competition with other variant interpretations? Presumably, a few alternatives assemble in parallel until one gains the strong "legs" needed to allow it to become robust enough to establish hegemony. If the *leave* link stumbles, the *saw* hexagons might not compete very effectively, and so the top level dangles.

That's stratified stability at work, and it may be what enables a series of simple rules, at the level of argument structure, to generate a proper syntax. Each verb has a characteristic set of links: some required, some optional, some prohibited. The conglomeration is called a sentence if all the obligatory links are satisfied and no words are left dangling, unsupported by a structural role.

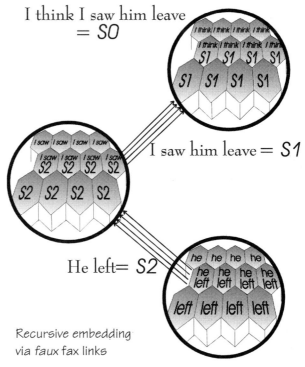

I think I saw him leave $= S0$

I saw him leave $= S1$

He left $= S2$

Recursive embedding via faux fax links

A sentence tells a little story with characteristic roles. Most verbs require a subject-actor-agent but it can be a noun phrase such as *The tall blond man with one black shoe* or even a sentence itself such as *What you see*). Beyond that near generality, special cases abound. The intransitive verb *sleep* cannot tolerate an object-patient-theme (*He sleeps it* is a clanger). The verb *give* insists on both a recipient and an item given. I discuss such required and optional roles at more length in *How Brains Think* and suggest a mechanistic analogy for how such argument structure operates.

So the "meaning of the sentence" is, in this model, an abstract cerebral code whose hexagons compete for territory with those suggesting alternative interpretations. Phrase structure is presumably a matter of the coherent corticocortical links to contributing territories, having their own competitions and tendencies to die out if not reinforced by backprojecting codes. Weblike crosstalk between subchoruses presumably occurs, and may be quite useful so long as it remains weak enough not to show up on the audit trail. Argument structure suggests multilobed attractors (p. 155).

Surface structure, needed to actually speak one word after another, is a matter of unpacking the contributors in an order commensurate with a particular language's surface structure conventions. The 18-to-36-month-old child seems to tune up this circuitry for the patterns of a particular language without much overt trial-and-error, merely by listening to the speech of others. In English, they include a subject-verb-object word order for simple declarative sentences, to which you add the inflections for plurals or tense, and perhaps some case markings (such as he-him, who-whom) to provide the listener with additional clues about whether the noun plays a subject or object role in the verb's story.

So COHERENT CORTICOCORTICALS buy you some essentials of phrase structure via a colonizing choir. What might degrade such a nice system into a protolanguage? Incoherence will do. Were the corticocortical's error correction not well tuned, linkages would be restricted to well-practiced special cases, perhaps only the spatiotemporal firing patterns for a limited number of vocabulary items, perhaps a few schemas and scripts.

That's because a cerebral code for an item is no longer the same, here and there. Jumble and smear means that a muddled version must be gradually learned by the target cortex; if sent back, a doubly-distorted version must be learned and an equivalence constructed to the original. The return path would be slow and chancy, and it is what allows a subchorus to be maintained and thereby permits an audit trail to resolve ambiguities. Lacking such structure would be very limiting, like signal flags on sailing ships, giving you a small shared vocabulary with only minor possibilities for novel associations. Embedding would probably be restricted to stock phrases. Relating who did what to whom would take a long time — just as in "protolanguage."

Adding *faux* faxing to a base that included regional darwinian copying competitions, each using memorized relationships to shape up quality, is thus a candidate for what made proto-language into Language Itself. Corticocortical coherence that became good enough to convey even arbitrary spatiotemporal patterns could have implemented the recursive embedding and long-range links aspects of Universal Grammar — and have done it in one step, without semistructured intermediate forms.

Though there is much for linguists and archaeologists to sort out, some now think that a big language step accompanied the evolution of *Homo erectus* to early *Homo sapiens* about a quarter-million years ago. The arbitrary cerebral code linkages described here, in the context of a Darwin Machine at each end to augment quality, might provide the improved capabilities needed to convert the infrequently innovating *Homo erectus* culture (a million years of stasis) into our prolific one, capable of occasionally producing the incandescent mind of a Plato or Shakespeare.

THERE EMERGES FROM THIS VIEW OF OUR BRAIN, with its relentless rearrangement from moment to moment, some glimpses of the neural foundations on which we construct our utterances and think our thoughts, some suggestions for how thoughts might miscue, and some possibilities for implementing the shortcut rules which make possible our kind of language and rational thought.

Since Darwin's recognition of how biology could have been bootstrapped by natural selection operating on inherited variation, the immune response has been recognized as more than just an analogy: rather, it's the same *process*, operating on the intermed-iate time scale of days to weeks (though running out of gas as the antigen is eliminated). By now, I think that we can recognize a darwinian process per se, what I have called a Darwin Machine, capable of operating on various time scales and in various media able to reproduce with inherited variation, as one of the key org-anizing principles of the universe. In the brain, such a process need not run out of challenges, as memes from a rich cultural life always provide another set of complex patterns to analyze for possible hidden structure, repeating the process that we used as two-year-olds to figure out the syntax of the utterances we heard.

The extensive parallelism between Darwin's 1859 formulation of principles, and the ones now suggested for hexagonal cloning competitions on the milliseconds-to-minutes time scale, can easily be seen by paraphrasing Darwin's final paragraph of *On the Origin of Species* so as to emphasize the power of this process as it could be manifested in cerebral cortex. And borrowing Darwin's finale framework seems only appropriate: it is, after all, his process.

IT IS INTERESTING TO CONTEMPLATE a tangled mind, clothed with memories of many kinds, with prototypical birds singing on the hallucinated bushes, with various thoughts flitting about, and with wormlike obsessions crawling through the damp cortex, and to reflect that these elaborately constructed forms, so different from each other, and dependent upon each other in so complex a manner, have all been produced by laws acting around us. These laws, taken in the largest sense, being Reproduction via clones of cerebral codes; Variability from their interdigitation and escapes from error correction, and from use and disuse; Inheritance which follows from surface-to-volume principles at the perimeter of cloned territories; a Ratio of Increase so high as to lead to a Struggle for cortical space, and as a consequence to Natural Selection from current and memorized environments, entailing Divergence of Character and the Extinction of less-improved forms. Thus, from the war of random thoughts initially no better than those of our nighttime dreams, the most exalted process which we are capable of conceiving, namely, the production of the higher thoughts, directly follows. There is grandeur in this view of mental life, with its ascending powers. From such a darwinian ratchet for creating and refining ever more complex levels of abstraction, there arose unbidden our own brain of unbounded potential, able to discover the syntactic rules that nestle sentences within sentences, able to invent new rules that extend mere narratives into the long chains of rational thought. Transcending its origins in tool use and social life, our reorganized brain can now use stratified stability to explore the endless realm of memes. Blind to our foundations, we nonetheless created poetry and reason; with a clearer footing, we can perhaps contemplate how our heightened consciousness evolved and is evolving.

It is interesting to contemplate a tangled bank, clothed with many plants of many kinds, with birds singing on the bushes, with various insects flitting about, and with worms crawling through the damp earth, and to reflect that these elaborately constructed forms, so different from each other, and dependent upon each other in so complex a manner, have all been produced by laws acting around us. These laws, taken in the largest sense, being Growth with Reproduction; Inheritance which is almost implied by reproduction; Variability from the indirect and direct action of the conditions of life and from use and disuse: a Ratio of Increase so high as to lead to a Struggle for Life, and as a consequence to Natural Selection, entailing Divergence of Character and the Extinction of less-improved forms. Thus, from the war of nature, from famine and death, the most exalted object which we are capable of conceiving, namely, the production of the higher animals, directly follows. There is grandeur in this view of life, with its several powers, having been originally breathed by the Creator into a few forms or into one; and that, whilst this planet has gone cycling on according to the fixed law of gravity, from so simple a beginning endless forms most beautiful and most wonderful have been, and are being evolved.

CHARLES DARWIN, 1859

Afterthoughts

I thank Jennifer S. Lund for introducing me to the properties of the intrinsic horizontal connections of neocortex, and for regularly attempting to straighten out my misconceptions. David G. King was heroic, marking up two versions of the manuscript from his unique viewpoint in both population biology and local circuit neurobiology, and suggesting I emphasize that variation need not be truly random. Stephen Jay Gould kindly looked over the six darwinian essentials and suggested emphasizing Darwin's inheritance principle. Theodore H. Bullock, Walter J. Freeman, and Dan Downs were most helpful in their comments on the finished manuscript, as was Katherine Graubard in the preceding four years. Mac Wells managed to sketch most of my wild ideas for text illustrations and cartoons, and Mark Meyer did the wonderful painting "Hexacode" for the cover. Doug vanderHoof and Mark Crawford labored mightily to get an author portrait. I thank them all, together with Fiona Stevens, Amy Pierce, and Michael Rutter at MIT Press.

Many neuroscientists can trace their scientific roots back to the pioneers via only several generations of mentors. Mine go back to Donald Hebb via Steve Glickman, now professor of psychology at Berkeley, who, when I was a physics undergraduate at Northwestern in the late 1950s and he was the closest thing to a neuroscientist on campus, told me about how Hebb posed the important problems and arranged for me to visit Montreal. My relevant roots also go back to Keffer Hartline and the lateral inhibition problem via his student Chuck Stevens, with whom I subsequently did my Ph.D. thesis a few years later in Seattle.

So, I was in possession of most of the essential components of the problem long before a solution finally coalesced in 1991, all thanks to the way others had formulated the problems they studied, even when they couldn't solve them. The missing key was the "dog that didn't bark in the night," those silent sidestepping gaps that pattern the recurrent excitation, that Jenny Lund told me about in 1991. No wonder that everything fell together so rapidly thereafter.

allele   Alternate forms of a gene. Perhaps 20 percent of your expressed genes have a different allele on the other chromosome, that is, you are *heterozygous* for that gene and might switch to using it under some conditions. One reason that hybrids don't breed true to type is that parents are often passing on their less-used allele. Inbred strains have less heterozygosity. [18, 103, 140]

area   When capitalized, it's a Brodmann Area, a subdivision of cerebral cortex based on the relative thickness of the six layers. Area 17 is better known as primary visual cortex; it seems to be a functional unit but Area 19 comprises at least six major functional units. A **territory** or **work space** is an area occupied temporarily by active patterns of cloned hexagons.

attractor   If you plot one variable against another for a series of times, the successive points may seem to move along a trajectory, often a cyclical one. This *phase portrait* may well look like an oddly-shaped orbit around an imaginary gravitational attractor, from whence the name. All of my chaotic illustrations are in such a *phase space*. There are four general classes of attractors: point (say, the neuron's resting state), periodic (as in pacemaker cells), quasi-periodic, and chaotic. The magnets in my loopy illustrations serve as a stand-in for a quasi-periodic attractor, as would an organ pipe. Whereas pipes have well-defined harmonics, chaotic attractors have overtones everywhere, in the manner of white noise. Chaotic systems are highly sensitive to initial conditions; while somewhat predictable in the short run, they may do surprising things in the long run. [66]

automatic gain control (AGC)   A process that reduces gain (loudness, in a typical auditory application) as input levels increase. It tends to make the output levels about the same for faint and loud inputs — unless the faint one occurs soon after the loud one, as it takes time for the gain to be raised again. The nineteenth-century speed governor for engines was an example of an AGC, and modern tape recorders use them. [77]

axon   The neuron's "wire," a long (0.1 - 2,000 mm), spiderthread-thin portion of the neuron that carries voltages between the neuron's input sites (concentrated on cell body and dendritic tree) and the neuron's outputs, its many-branched axon terminals that make synapses onto downstream neurons. It's typically a one-way street, messages flowing from the dendrites and cell body to the far end of the axon where synapses are made. [26, 31, 34]

basin of attraction   If one thinks of the attractor as the low point of a washbowl, then starting points on the counter top lie outside the basin of attraction. Starting anywhere within the basin results in a trajectory that circles around the attractor. Basins can be discontinuous, as seen in pinball games. A *bifurcation* is a change from one basin of attraction to another, in the manner of changing gaits. [68]

binding   In linguistics, binding is the part of the grammar which determines the reference of such words as *he, himself, each other*. In cognitive neuroscience, binding is the notion that some process must maintain links between the various features of a perceived object during cognitive processing, given the dispersal of object features to those *what* specialists in temporal lobe and to the *where* aspects specialists up in parietal areas. One simple proposal is that the involved neurons in these dispersed areas actually become synchronized, and that this is what recouples *red* with the top light on the traffic signal (another object's features — say, those characterizing the approaching pedestrian — synchronize at different times). This proposed use of synchrony is, of course, on a much grander scale than I propose for the triangular arrays, which might span a few millimeters. Binding may not be needed except for very complex sensory scenes, such as the streaming encountered when brachiating through the trees or driving a car; some suspect that the perceived need for binding to reassemble specialists is a remnant of the cartesian theater reasoning that Dennett critiques. [56]

bottleneck   An evolutionary event that greatly narrows the variability in a population. [93]

cell-assembly   Donald O. Hebb's 1949 coinage for a group of cortical neurons that subserves and sustains the active memory trace that follows perception. [104]

central nervous system (CNS)   The brain, spinal cord, and the retina (all the rest is the peripheral nervous system).

cerebral cortex The outer 2 mm (that's two thin coins worth) of the brain's cerebral hemispheres with a layered structure. It isn't required for performing a lot of simple actions but seems essential for creating new episodic memories, the fancier associations, and many new movement programs. *Paleocortex* (*archicortex*) such as hippocampus has a simpler structure and earlier evolutionary appearance than the six-plus-layered *neocortex*. [29]

chaos   Complicated patterns that are not truly random. Chaos is a cryptic form of order, what a random-number generator produces.

There is, as the phrase goes, "a sensitive dependence on initial conditions." Because chaos was defined in a paradoxical way ("It may look random, but it's merely *chaotic*"), it is a term often misused or misunderstood. See **attractor, basin of attraction, itinerancy**.

chunking Collapsing multiple-word phrases into a single one, in the manner of acronyms.

cipher A disguising transformation of a message without using chunking, such as a simple substitution cipher.

code In cryptography, a disguising transformation that also chunks — and thereby shortens — the message, as when a number stands for a standard five-word phrase. More generally, as in genetic code, it refers to the transformation of a representation's short form into its long-form implementation. As such, it is analogous to a matrix. It may also simply refer to the short form itself, such as a DNA base-pair sequence capable of generating a particular protein.

columns A minicolumn is a cylindrical group of about 100 neurons extending through all the layers of neocortex and about 0.030 mm in diameter, usually organized around a dendritic bundle; the orientation column is an example. Macrocolumns are a hundred times larger in area (and about 0.5 mm across) and often more like curtain folds than cylinders; they are typically identified by common inputs, e.g., the ocular dominance columns of visual cortex. [42]

corticocortical connection An axon or axon bundle connecting one patch of cerebral cortex to another. Some remain local, within the superficial layers of cortex, while others go through the white matter to distant targets — some, via the corpus callosum, to the other cerebral hemisphere. See photograph, p. 131.

Darwin Machine My 1987 coinage, on the Turing Machine analogy, for any full-fledged darwinian process incorporating the six essentials for the darwinian algorithm. Species evolution, the immune response, some genetic algorithms, and the hexagonal work space competitions are all examples.

deme A geographic subpopulation, mostly inbreeding but with occasional gene flow via migrants from the larger metapopulation.

dendrite Neurons have branches. There is a single thin **axon** that initiates and propagates impulses to distant destinations, and there are somewhat thicker dendritic branches that receive synapses from other neurons's axon terminals. Pyramidal neurons have a tall-tree-like *apical dendrite* plus some rootlike *basal dendrites*. At least in neocortex, dendrites are the receiving branches of the neuron and the axon is the sending branch. Elsewhere, some dendrites can also act like axon terminals, releasing neurotransmitter in response to impulses and local voltage changes. [26, 31]

efference copy   The notion that, in generating movement commands, the nervous system also generates an expected set of sensory inputs that will result from the movement, the comparison of expected and actual serving to warn of problems in the execution of the movement.

empty niche   A proven *niche* space that is temporarily unoccupied by a tenant species.

error correction   Schemes that detect (in the manner of checksums) but also correct transmission errors using some form of redundancy; commonly used in tape backups.

faux **fax**   My coinage for a faxlike telecopying process, one that reproduces a spatiotemporal pattern some distance away.

gene   A unit of heredity, essentially that segment of a DNA molecule comprising the code for a particular peptide or protein. We also talk loosely of "a gene for blue eyes" and so forth, but many a DNA gene is pleiotropic: it has multiple (and sometimes very different) effects on its body. As for what's a unit, here's Helena Cronin's answer:

> The answer must be: When it's a unit that selection can work on . . . a gene and the ramifying tree of all its phenotypic effects (in comparison with alternative forms of the gene, its alleles). If it should turn out that the bone of a toe and the shape of an eyebrow are pleiotropic effects of the same gene, then that bizarre combination is a respectable adaptive unit. Natural selection works on genetic differences in populations. If a genetic change that lengthens the bone also curves the eyebrow, then our adaptive explanation should recognize that; we should be interested in the genetic differences that give rise not merely to differences in toe-length but to differences in toe-length-plus-eyebrow-shape, even if eyebrow shape should turn out to be selectively neutral. This is an answer that would not have been obvious to the organism-centered view of classical Darwinism but comes readily to a theory that is gene-centered.

gene repertoires   When alternative forms of a gene are expressed at different stages of development, e.g., fetal hemoglobin is replaced by the adult version.

genetic code   A table with 4^3 (64) entries that tells you which of the 20 amino acids will result from a particular triplet of the four types of RNA nucleotides, e.g., CAU yields histidine (as does CAC).

genotype   The full set of genes carried by an individual, whether expressed or silent alleles. Similar to *genome*. Compare to *phenotype*.

What makes living matter so different from other self-organizing systems is that a cell has an information center, the genes, concerned with orchestrating the many different processes going on within the cell, and in such a manner that copies of the cell tend to survive.

grammar, universal   Each of the languages of the world has a corresponding mental grammar, constructed as we learn the language. Though they differ in many ways, the human brain seems to have a highly specific menu of possibilities for grammatical organization, known as Universal Grammar, or UG, that structures language learning even when the input itself is lacking in structure (pidgins, home sign, and so on). See JACKENDOFF (1993).

hash   A hash is a unique short-form identifier, a "fingerprint" of something more complicated. One simple application is to create a file name that isn't already in use — and also isn't unnecessarily long, since you want a low-dimensional search space that can be scanned rapidly. Using the seconds and minutes fields of file modification time stamps often suffices for a hash; a document can also be hashed by using the least significant bits of a checksum.

Hebbian synapse   Hebb proposed that a successful synapse is strengthened: "When an axon of cell A is near enough [the synaptic cleft hadn't yet been seen in 1949] to excite cell B and repeatedly or persistently takes part in firing it, some growth process or metabolic change takes place in one or both cells such that A's efficiency, as one of the cells firing B, is increased."

immune response   Following infection with an antigen, a process begins that gradually destroys the foreign molecules — but, in the process lasting days to weeks, the initially inefficient antibodies evolve into much better fits to the antigen. Because they linger in the body for some time, immunity to further infection is achieved.

impulse   *Action potential* and *spike* are synonyms; it's the regenerative change in the voltage across the neuron's membrane used for long-distance (more than a millimeter) signaling in the nervous system. It is brief (1/1000 sec, quicker than any other signal in the brain but a million times slower than computers) and large (only 1/10 volt but bigger than any other voltage in the brain). Its threshold property can also be used as a simple decision making mechanism. See also **axon, myelin, sodium channel**.

in vitro   "In glass" is used to designate experiments carried out in a dish on cells that have been removed from their natural setting. [3]

in situ   "as situated" is (along with *in vivo*) the opposite of *in vitro*.
[3]

inheritance principle   Darwin's great but often misunderstood insight, that variation is not truly random. Rather than variations being done from some ideal or average type, small undirected variations are preferentially done from the more successful individuals of the current generation, exploring the solution space nearby (not jumping randomly to somewhere truly unrelated) in the next generation. [21, 101]

interneuron   An "insider neuron." Most CNS neurons are interneurons; the only ones which aren't are the sensory neurons and the motor neurons that drive the muscles. An interneuron receives input from about 2,000-10,000 "upstream" neurons and transmits its output to a similar number of "downstream" neurons — occasionally even one of its own input neurons, creating a loop (see figure, p. 32).

ion   An atom or small free-floating molecule with a net electrical charge. When NaCl dissolves in water, most of its weak chemical bonds break, but the Cl carries away one of the Na's electrons, and so they become the ions Cl^- and Na^+. The major players in the extracellular space outside the neuron's membrane are Ca^{++}, Cl^- and Na^+, with much of the K^+ concentrated inside cells. The Ca^{++} inside cells tends to be tightly regulated ("buffered") by various mechanisms because it too can serve a signal function (a "second messenger," the first being the neurotransmitter) for the slower processes that follow synaptic transmission.

island biogeography   The peculiarities of animal and plant species when largely isolated, with just occasional interbreeding. An "island" can also be a deep ocean basin, a high mountain valley, or a patch in a patchy resource distribution that prevents migration. Islands often have a reduced number of species, so traditional predators or parasites may be lacking. Species often arrive in small numbers, so bottlenecks are a standard feature of island populations.

itinerancy   Like the seasonal progress of a peddler revisiting towns that have changed somewhat since the last visit, chaotic itinerancy emphasizes the recurrence of similar, rather than identical, states. [120]

limit cycle   A type of nonlinear oscillator, such as a threshold device with reset (cisterns that automatically flush when refilled).

linkage   In genetics, an association between the expression of two gene alleles that is greater than could be expected from random assortment. For example, two adjacent genes may tend to move together during meiosis.

long-term potentiation (LTP)   A sustained (minutes to days) change in connection strength, largely synaptic, that follows some priming events — such as a barrage of impulses. Originally seen via conditioning and testing in the same pathway, it has also been seen to cross over from separate conditioning and test pathways. LTP is thought to provide the physiological scaffolding for slowly making (during memory consolidation) the anatomical changes that more permanently increase the synaptic strength. [75]

meiosis   The cell division used for making sperm and ova (as compared to ordinary *mitosis*), notable for the crossing-over of chromosomes that results in a shuffling of the grandparents' genes and for the reduction of diploid to haploid.

meme   Richard Dawkins's 1976 coinage, on the analogy to gene (with a little aid from mime and mimic), for a cultural copying unit, such as the word or melody that is mimicked by others.

membrane   All cells are a bag of components, separated from the extracellular fluid and other cells by a limiting membrane. There are transport systems within this membrane, little pumps throwing sodium ions out of the cell while bringing potassium ions into the cell. There are ion channels through the membrane, pores that allow certain sizes of ions (and therefore certain types) to move inside and out. A channel may be controlled by a receptor-guarded gate on the external surface (the typical neurotransmitter-activated route for producing current flows), by the electrical field across the membrane (the typical voltage-gated channels that produce the impulse), or sometimes both (see **NMDA**).

memory, dual trace   Hebb's 1949 coinage for separate systems implementing short- and long-term memories: active (spatiotemporal) and passive (spatial-only) memory traces.

memory, episodic   One-trial learning involving distinct episodes, such as being an eyewitness to an accident. Such memories are notoriously malleable, influenced by subsequent events and the mistakes made in recall attempts.

message digest   The fingerprintlike result of a computation (see **hash**) that reduces a long document to a number that serves to uniquely characterize it; were any changes to be made in the document — even adding an extra space — a different message digest would result. Although you cannot reconstruct the document from the message digest, nor does it serve as an abstract, you can use it for recognition ("I've seen exactly this before"). [17]

metapopulation   A population with dispersed demes that replenish one another with migrants.

myelin   Some of the longer axon branches are insulated with myelin (whose fat content is what gives the white matter its characteristic color), flat layers of which are wrapped around the axon in the manner of a bandage roll. This reduces the electrical capacitance that the impulse must charge up (the old capacitors-in-series trick), thereby speeding impulse propagation. The sodium channels that open during the upstroke of an impulse are confined to unwrapped axon regions, little exposed gaps called *nodes of Ranvier*, thereby reducing the metabolic cleanup costs by confining them to the small percentage of unwrapped axon cylinder. Without myelin, the impulse slowly spreads in the manner of a burning fuse; with myelin, the impulse seemingly jumps from one node to the next (saltatory conduction), achieving conduction speeds a hundred-fold greater than seen in unmyelinated conduction, top speeds being about 150 mm/msec.

neocortex   All of cerebral cortex except for *archicortex* (olfactory cortex, hippocampus), the simpler layered structure that lacks the patterned recurrent excitatory connections and columnar structures which make the six-layered neocortex so interesting. [29]

nervous system   The whole works, both central nervous system (CNS: brain, spinal cord, and retinas) and peripheral nervous system (most sensory and muscle connections, plus the clusters of neurons called ganglia).

neuromodulator   A molecule traversing the synaptic cleft to bind at a postsynaptic receptor site is acting as a **neurotransmitter** but it can also act as a neuromodulator (affecting the responsiveness to other neurotransmitters), typically by affecting internal processes in the downstream neuron over a longer time scale; it need not travel via the synaptic cleft, but might diffuse like a local hormone from release sites in the neighborhood. The major diffusely broadcasting systems for norepinephrine, acetylcholine, dopamine, and serotonin from subcortical regions surely involve profound neuromodulator actions in neocortex, quite in addition to their more immediate neuro-transmitter effects.

neuron   The nerve cell, whether sensory neuron, interneuron, or motor neuron. There are about 10^{12} neurons in the human brain and spinal cord; the neocortex alone is said to have 10^{11}. The *cell body* of the neuron is the widest section (see figure, p. 26), thanks to containing the cell nucleus, and there are many processes branching off, receiving inputs and distributing outputs. See **dendrite, axon**.

neurotransmitter A molecule such as glutamate or acetylcholine that is released from an axon terminal (often by the arrival of an **impulse**), diffuses across a narrow extracellular space, and binds with a receptor on the surface of the **postsynaptic** cell. Many dozens of neurotransmitters have been identified over the years, and a given axon terminal may release more than one kind.

niche The "outward projection of the needs of an organism" such as food resources, camouflage from predators, suitable housing and sites for effective reproduction.

NMDA The NMDA channel at glutamate synapses was, unfortunately, named after N-methyl-D-aspartate because that molecule, rather than glutamate, is what opens the postsynaptic channel in the lowest doses. But glutamate opens it almost as well, and that's what is usually released as a neurotransmitter. The real significance of an NMDA synapse is that the current state of the dendrite's voltage, at the time the neurotransmitter arrives, is also important: Mg^{++} tends to plug the channels through the membrane, blocking Na^+ and Ca^{++} inflows, but an antecedent rise in dendritic voltage (whether from the same synapse or neighbors) will unplug some such channels, allowing a much larger response. This is a major source of dendritic amplification of synaptic currents, along with the persistent sodium channels in the apical dendrites, and an example of what Hebb predicted in 1949 (see **Hebbian synapse**).

node The theoretical term for an intersection in one of my triangular arrays. In the anatomy, it corresponds to a single superficial pyramidal neuron (or perhaps to a minicolumn of act-alike neurons). [40]

parcellation Fragmentation; breaking apart a population into smaller, isolated units ("parcels"). Rising sea level converts a hilly island into an archipelago.

phenotype Usually "body" but actually the entire constitution of an individual (anatomical, physiological, behavioral) resulting from the interaction of the genes with the environment. As Dawkins emphasized in *The Extended Phenotype*, it can even grade into things such as bird nests.

postsynaptic The postsynaptic neuron's dendrite receives neurotransmitter, rather in the manner of sniffing perfume, and changes the permeability of its membrane to certain ions, usually Na^+, K^+, Cl^-, or

Ca^{++} in some combination. The ion flows through the membrane in turn produce the voltage change known as the *postsynaptic potential* (PSP). If excitatory, it is called the EPSP; if inhibitory, the IPSP.

pyramidal neurons The excitatory neurons of neocortex. They typically have a tall apical dendrite (an exception is the spiny stellate neuron) and a triangular-shaped cell body (from whence the name), from which their axon leaves. The neurons contributing to the pyramidal tract (alias the corticospinal tract, named for the triangular shape of the axon bundle as it traverses the medulla) are themselves pyramidal neurons, but most pyramidal neurons send axons elsewhere. [26]

receptive field A map of the inputs to a single neuron, e.g., those parts of the skin of the hand that produce excitation or inhibition of a cortical neuron (antagonistic surrounds are especially common). The limited view of the world as seen by a single neuron. [28]

recombination There are several connotations: (1) The shuffling of genetic material between an individual's two chromosome pairs that occurs just prior to the production of ova or sperm (the crossing-over phase of meiosis) and (2) the production of a new individual through the union of a sperm and an ovum from two parents at fertilization.

recruitment In neurophysiology, this means getting other neurons to join the action, much as the expert choir "recruits" the audience in the *Hallelujah Chorus.*

resonance A relationship between two periodically moving bodies (say, two pendulum clocks on a shelf) in which their cycles eventually become locked together ("in sync," though often one cycle is some multiple of the other). More abstractly, a moving body may resonate with the stationary bumps in the road, or two chemical processes may resonate with one another and thereby synchronize their cycles. [65]

sodium channel A pore through the membrane of a size to admit hydrated Na^+ but not most other ions, controlled by gating mechanisms near the outer surface that open when the trans-membrane voltage is becoming less negative. This admits even more Na^+, making the inside even less negative. When these currents exceed those of counterbalancing outward potassium currents (this occurs at a voltage called the *threshold*), you get a regenerative cycle continuing for a hundred millivolt rise, known as the **impulse**. More sluggish mechanisms on the inner surface tend to close the channel opening, and thereby help (along with potassium entry through other voltage-sensitive channels) to terminate the impulse and create a *refractory period* of several milliseconds in which it is more difficult to initiate another impulse.

schema   As in "schematic outline," it's a mental item more abstract than a rich mental image of an object. In some cognitive contexts, it is used more narrowly for those things like *more, less, bigger, inside* — things grounded in our everyday experiences, often making reference to our own body moving through our daily world. Movements need something similar, and schema is often used to refer to standard movement programs. [161]

spine, dendritic   A small protrusion, like a thorn, on the shaft of a **dendrite** that receives several synaptic contacts from presynaptic **axons**. See figure on p. 26.

stellate neurons   The other general class of neurons in the neocortex, on the basis of anatomy.   Physiologically, most of them have inhibitory actions, an exception being the spiny stellates.

synapse   The synapse is the junction between neurons across which communications flow, usually in the form of *neurotransmitter* molecules secreted by the *presynaptic* axon terminal that diffuse a short distance across the extracellular space (the *synaptic cleft*) to the *postsynaptic* neuron, on whose membrane are some receptor molecules to which the neurotransmitter molecules reversibly bind. While they are bound, they open up an ion channel through the postsynaptic membrane, producing postsynaptic current flow. Most drugs affecting the CNS operate by interfering with synaptic transmission. See also **dendrite, Hebbian synapse, neuromodulator, neurotransmitter, NMDA, postsynaptic, spine.** [26]

threshold   The word has two connotations in neurophysiology, one of which has a lot of imprecise reciprocals. As used in describing the **sodium channel**, the threshold is the transmembrane voltage (say, -56 mV) at which the inward and outward currents are in unstable equilibrium and above which the inward current becomes regenerative (the upstroke of the impulse). But a "high threshold" is also used in the same way as saying "low excitability," that you've got, say, 20 mV to go from -76 mV before triggering an impulse. The phrase doesn't imply that the threshold voltage has risen to, say, -40 mV. My sea level metaphor for the AGC is based on this latter use: increased sea level is a stand-in for lower gain which would decrease the chances of exceeding threshold.

Recommended Reading

FREDERICK DAVID ABRAHAM with RALPH H. ABRAHAM, CHRISTOPHER D. SHAW, *A Visual Introduction to Dynamical Systems Theory for Psychology* (Aerial Press, Santa Cruz 1990).

DEREK BICKERTON, *Language and Thought* (University of Washington Press 1995).

WILLIAM H. CALVIN, *How Brains Think* (BasicBooks 1996).

WILLIAM H. CALVIN, *The Cerebral Symphony* (Bantam 1989).

WILLIAM H. CALVIN and GEORGE A. OJEMANN, *Conversations with Neil's Brain: The Neural Nature of Thought and Language* (Addison-Wesley 1994).

HELENA CRONIN, *The Ant and the Peacock* (Cambridge University Press 1991).

DANIEL C. DENNETT, *Darwin's Dangerous Idea* (Simon & Schuster 1995).

GERALD M. EDELMAN, *The Remembered Present* (BasicBooks 1989).

WALTER J. FREEMAN, *Societies of Brains* (Erlbaum 1995).

LEON GLASS and MICHAEL C. MACKEY, *From Clocks to Chaos: The Rhythms of Life* (Princeton University Press 1988).

DONALD O. HEBB, *Essay on Mind* (Erlbaum 1980).

J. ALLAN HOBSON, *The Chemistry of Conscious States: How the Brain Changes its Mind* (Little, Brown 1994).

RAY JACKENDOFF, *Patterns in the Mind: Language and Human Nature* (BasicBooks 1993).

MARK JOHNSON, *The Body in the Mind* (University of Chicago Press 1987).

MARVIN MINSKY, *The Society of Mind* (Simon & Schuster 1986).

OLAF SPORNS and GIULIO TONINI, editors, *Selectionism and the Brain* (Academic Press 1994; also appears as volume 37 of the *International Review of Neurobiology*).

IAN STEWART, *Nature's Numbers* (BasicBooks 1995).

Notes

Because good medical libraries are few and far between, I have attempted to cite the most widely available articles and books (though I often have to cite specialty journals instead). Short-form citations such as DENNETT (1995) either refer to a book in my *Recommended Reading* list or to a nearby full-length citation.

Prologue

page

1 STEPHEN JAY GOULD, *Ontogeny and Phylogeny* (Harvard University Press 1977).

1 See the last chapter of JEAN PIAGET, *Le langage et la pensee chez l'enfant* (Neuchatel 1923).

3 This use of *code* subsumes the more common uses of *neural code*, e.g., those referring to firing rate, spike timing, etc., all of which are derivative of the 1950's auditory *place* versus *frequency* code debates. Code often just means representation or mapping. For some modern discussion, see

TERRENCE J. SEJNOWSKI, "Time for a new neural code?" *Nature* 376:21-22 (6 July 1995);

JOHN J. HOPFIELD, "Pattern recognition computation using action potential timing for stimulus representation," *Nature* 376:33-36 (6 July 1995);

SAM A. DEADWYLER and ROBERT E. HAMPSON, "Ensemble activity and behavior: what's the code?" *Science* 270:1316-1318 (24 November 1995);

A. P. GEORGOPOULOS, A. ASHE, N. SMYRNIS, M. TAIRA, "The motor cortex and the coding of force," *Science* 256: 1692-1695 (1992).

4 KENNETH J. W. CRAIK, *The Nature of Explanation* (Cambridge University Press 1943), p. 61.

4 DENNETT (1995).

4 WILLIAM H. CALVIN, "The brain as a Darwin Machine," *Nature* 330:33-34 (5 November 1987).

4 William James's development of his darwinian theory of mind, see pp. 433ff of ROBERT J. RICHARDS, *Darwin and the Emergence of Evolutionary Theories of Mind and Behavior* (University of Chicago Press 1987).

4 Other examples of darwinian processes include so-called "genetic algorithms" in computer science and molecular biology techniques seen in the RNA evolution experiments. See

JOHN H. HOLLAND, "Genetic algorithms," *Scientific American* 267(1):66-72 (July 1992).

GERALD F. JOYCE, "Directed molecular evolution," *Scientific American* 267(6):90-97 (December 1992).

5   LUDWIG WITTGENSTEIN, *Philosophical Investigations* (Basil Blackwell 1953).

5   J. ALLAN HOBSON, *The Dreaming Brain* (Basic Books 1988).

5   CHARLES DARWIN, *On the Origin of Species* (1859).

6   "...most "darwinian" discussions...." See articles in SPORNS AND TONINI (1994).

6   The background is in WILLIAM H. CALVIN, "Islands in the mind: dynamic subdivisions of association cortex and the emergence of a Darwin Machine," *Seminars in the Neurosciences* 3(5):423-433 (1991). WILLIAM H. CALVIN, ``The emergence of intelligence,'' *Scientific American* 271(4):100-107 (October 1994; also appears in the Scientific American book *Life in the Universe*, 1995 -- N.B., the hexagons figure is an editorial error; simply ignore it or see the web page for the unaltered version: *http://weber.u.washington.edu/~wcalvin/sciamer.html*

6   This book-length consideration of the issues was delayed by several other books in progress, though I did manage some brief treatments, e.g., in the last chapter of *Conversations with Neil's Brain* and in the latter half of my *Scientific American* article. Chapter 7 of *How Brains Think* summarizes my neocortical Darwin Machine scheme but *The Cerebral Code* is its first complete description.

7   Charles Ives, see p. 366 of JOSEPH MACHLIS, *The Enjoyment of Music*, "5th ed. shorter" (W. W. Norton 1984).

8   Mac Wells illustrated my archaeoastronomy book, *How the Shaman Stole the Moon* (Bantam 1991).

8   Simulations were half of my Ph.D. thesis, a means of seeing if observed noise could account for the actual stochastic interspike interval variability of cat spinal motor neurons. I have been skeptical of free-parameter curve-fitting that is hidden from view even of the simulation's proprietor ever since. See W. H. CALVIN and C. F. STEVENS, "Synaptic noise and other sources of randomness in motoneuron interspike intervals," *Journal of Neurophysiology* 31:574-587 (1968).

9   ERNST MAYR, "Population thinking and neuronal selection: metaphors or concepts?" In *Selectionism and the Brain*, edited by Olaf Sporns and Giulio Tonini (Academic Press 1994), pp.27-34 at p.29.

9   NIELS K. JERNE, "Antibodies and learning: Selection versus instruction," in *The Neurosciences: A Study Program*, edited by G. C. Quarton, T. Melnechuk, & F. O. Schmitt (Rockefeller University Press 1967), pp. 200-205 at p. 204.

Chapter 1.
The Representation Problem and the Copying Solution

11 ANTONIO R. DAMASIO, *Descartes' Error* (Putnam 1995), p.12.

11 Those aware of the philosophical battles over the word *representation* should realize that I'm always using it in the sense of a cerebral code, not an external symbol or sign. For a similar neurophysiologically-based perspective that bypasses unnecessary hangups, see FREEMAN (1995), pp. 106-108.

11 Christmas dinner quip: FREEMAN (1995), p.55.

13 Taste coding: ROBERT P. ERICKSON, "On the neural bases of behavior," *American Scientist* 72:233-241 (May-June 1984). An endnote in my *The Cerebral Symphony*, at p. 359, discusses its application to orientation-sensitive neurons of visual cortex with eighteen types of elementary templates.

13 IRVING KUPFERMAN, KENNETH R. WEISS, "The command neuron concept," *Behavioral and Brain Science* 1(1):3-39 (1978).

13 Schemas, see JOHNSON (1987).

13 DONALD O. HEBB, *The Organization of Behavior* (Wiley 1949). And see PETER M. MILNER, "The mind and Donald O. Hebb," *Scientific American* 268(1):124-129 (January 1993).

13 It is just as important that the other lights are off: indeed, it is well to occasionally recall that vertebrate photoreceptors have their maximum rate of neurotransmitter discharge in darkness; what the image of a star against the night star does is to create a local hole in a sea of photoreceptor activity. That this isn't necessarily seen at later stages of the visual pathway only testifies to the amount of spatial and temporal differencing that occurs in other layers of the retina.

14 Automata, see WILLIAM POUNDSTONE, *The Recursive Universe* (Morrow 1985).

15 HEBB (1949), p. 62.

16 Representations don't have to be codes, so long as they remain local. The withdrawal reflex is wired up so that various combinations of threatening stimuli get an appropriate set of motor neurons up and running. Yes, there's a representation of threat, but not necessarily a code in the sense of a cell-assembly of stereotyped pattern.

16 DONALD O. HEBB, *Essay on Mind* (Erlbaum 1980), epigram at p.1, history at p.81.

17 Predicting movements, see GEORGOPOULOS et al (1992).

17 PATRICIA S. GOLDMAN-RAKIC, "Working memory and the mind," *Scientific American* 267(3):73-79 (September 1992).

17   MOSHE ABELES, *Corticotonics: Neural Circuits of the Cerebral Cortex* (Cambridge University Press 1991).

E. VAADIA, I. HAALMAN, M. ABELES, H. BERGMAN, Y. PRUT, H. SLOVIN, A. AERTSEN, "Dynamics of neuronal interactions in monkey cortex in relation to behaviourial events," *Nature* 373:515-518 (9 February 1995).

18   ERWIN SCHRÖDINGER, *What is Life?* (Cambridge University Press 1944).

22   GERALD F. JOYCE, "Directed molecular evolution," *Scientific American* 267(6):90-97 (December 1992).

22   HOLLAND (1992).

23   There is potentially an enormous difference, in some species, between what's conceived and what survives *in utero* long enough to be born. In humans, only about one in five conceptions results in a term birth, suggesting that environmental factors could play a large role in biasing the characteristics of a human population.

24   "Lean mean machine...." CALVIN (1996).

24   A. M. LISTER, "Rapid dwarfing of red deer on Jersey in the last interglacial," *Nature* 342:539-542 (30 November 1989).

25   DARWIN (1859) writes in Chapter III:

> The number of humble-bees in any district depends in a great measure upon the number of field-mice, which destroy their combs and nests; and Col. Newman, who has long attended to the habits of humble-bees, believes that "more than two-thirds of them are thus destroyed all over England." Now the number of mice is largely dependent, as every one knows, on the number of cats; and Col. Newman says, "Near villages and small towns I have found the nests of humble-bees more numerous than elsewhere, which I attribute to the number of cats that destroy the mice." Hence it is quite credible that the presence of a feline animal in large numbers in a district might determine, through the intervention first of mice and then of bees, the frequency of certain flowers in that district!

25   JONATHAN WEINER, *The Beak of the Finch* (Knopf 1994).

25   *avoir l'esprit de l'escalier* is from HOWARD RHEINGOLD, *They Have a Word for It* (Tarcher 1987).

25   A female that selects a mate on the basis of quick mental performance in a male thereby augments the quickness of both her sons and (unless the gene is on the Y chromosome) daughters.

Chapter 2.   Cloning in Cerebral Cortex

For the local circuits of cerebral cortex, see the special issue of the journal *Cerebral Cortex* 3 (September/October 1993) edited by KATHLEEN S. ROCKLAND. An introduction to the iterated architecture aspects is

WILLIAM H. CALVIN, "Cortical columns, modules, and Hebbian cell assemblies," in *Handbook of Brain Theory and Neural Networks*, M. A. ARBIB, ed. (MIT Press 1995), pp. 269-272. Primary visual cortex is the best-studied area: JENNIFER S. LUND, "Anatomical organization of macaque monkey striate visual cortex," *Annual Reviews of Neuroscience* 11:253-288 (1988).

27 RICHARD DAWKINS, *The Selfish Gene* (Oxford University Press 1976).

28 Von Békésy's lateral inhibition experiments are recounted in FLOYD RATLIFF'S *Mach Bands: Quantitative Studies on Neural Networks in the Retina* (Holden-Day, San Francisco 1965).

28 C. STEPHANIS, HERBERT JASPER, "Recurrent collateral inhibition in pyramidal tract neurons," *Journal of Neurophysiology* 27:855-877 (1964).

28 R. J. DOUGLAS, C. KOCH, M. MAHOWALD, K. A. MARTIN, H. H. SUAREZ, "Recurrent excitation in neocortical circuits," *Science* 269:981-985 (18 August 1995).

31 It's not that the axons lack synapses in the "gaps" but that they have many-branched terminal trees clustering around the metric distance. See figure 3 of BARBARA A. MCGUIRE, CHARLES D. GILBERT, PATRICIA K. RIVLIN, TORSTEN N. WIESEL, "Targets of horizontal connections in macaque primary visual cortex," *Journal of Comparative Neurology* 305:370-392 (1991). Their Cell 1 is reproduced with permission in the present illustration.

31 R. A. FISKEN, L. J. GAREY, T. P. S. POWELL, "The intrinsic, association, and commissural connections of the visual cortex," *Philosophical Transactions of the Royal Society (London)* 272B:487-536 (1975).

31 The lattice connectivity in the superficial layers has been seen in all mammals examined except rats; even a marsupial, the quokka, has them (J. S. LUND, Seattle lecture, 27 February 1996).

31 GREG STUART, BERT SAKMANN, "Amplification of EPSPs by axo-somatic sodium channels in neocortical pyramidal neurons," *Neuron* 15:1065-1076 (November 1995).

32 A. DAS, CHARLES D. GILBERT, "Long-range horizontal connections and their role in cortical reorganization revealed by optical recording of cat primary visual cortex," *Nature* 375:780ff (29 June 1995). The inset illustration is a gray scale version of their color figure, as is the earlier "Mexican hat" figure.

32 ATSUSHI IRIKI, CONSTANTINE PAVLIDES, ASAF KELLER, HIROSHI ASANUMA, "Long-term potentiation of thalamic input to the motor cortex induced by coactivation of thalamocortical and corticocortical afferents," *Journal of Neurophysiology* 65:1435-1441 (1991).

32 RAFAEL LORENTE DE NÓ, "Analysis of the activity of the chains of internuncial neurons," *Journal of Neurophysiology* 1:207-244 (1938). Also see his article on cerebral cortex at pp. 288-315 in the 3d edition of John F. Fulton's *Physiology of the Nervous System*, Oxford University Press (1949).

32 ABELES (1991).

33 DAVID SOMERS and NANCY KOPELL, "Rapid synchronization through fast threshold modulation," *Biological Cybernetics* 68:393-407 (1993).

J. T. ENRIGHT, "Temporal precision in circadian systems: a reliable neuronal clock from unreliable components?" *Science* 209:1542-1544 (1980).

33 HUGH SMITH, "Synchronous flashing of fireflies," *Science* 82:51 (1935).

33 STEVEN STROGATZ, IAN STEWART, "Coupled oscillators and biological synchronization," *Scientific American* 269:102-109 (December 1993).

33 WOLF SINGER, "Synchronization of cortical activity and its putative role in information processing and learning," *Annual Review of Physiology* 55:349-374 (1993).

36 "Stepping connectivity" is a more general term than lattice, used to cover the instances where axons also terminate in stripes. The gaps and clusters are thought to be tuned up prenatally, perhaps secondary to the inhibitory actions of the large basket neurons of the superficial layers, whose axonal branches spread just wide enough to cover the gaps, but not so wide as to inhibit the next axon terminal path. If intermediate axon terminals were never successful during development because of countervailing inhibition, they might have been eliminated. The basic cluster and gap pattern of the superficial pyramidal neuron might therefore be secondary to that of the large basket neuron. The axons of the large basket neurons of the other layers do not spread widely enough to match the lattice spacing (and the ones in the rat are insufficient in all layers). See

JENNIFER S. LUND, TAKASHI YOSHIOKA, JONATHAN B. LEVITT, "Comparison of intrinsic connectivity in different areas of macaque monkey cerebral cortex," *Cerebral Cortex* 3:148-162 (March/April 1993).

37 Other organizing principles may well be at work, competing with perfect triangles. In primary visual cortex, for example, the orientation columns, color blobs, and ocular dominance factors may be pulling the clusters here and there.

Chapter 3. A Compressed Code Emerges

39 HEBB (1980), p. 88.

40 LUND et al. (1993).

41 E. RAUSELL, E. G. JONES, "Extent of intracortical arborization of thalamocortical axons as a determinant of representation in monkey somatic sensory cortex," *Journal of Neuroscience* 15:4270 (1995).

X. WANG, M. M. MERZENICH, K. SAMESHIMA, W. M. JENKINS, "Remodeling of hand representation in adult cortex determined by timing of tactile stimulation," *Nature* 378:71-75 (2 November 1995).

41 DANIEL Y. TS'O, R. D. FROSTIG, E. E. LIEKE, A. GRINVALD, "Functional organization of primate visual cortex revealed by high resolution optical imaging," *Science* 249:417-420 (27 July 1990).

41 WILLIAM H. CALVIN, PETER C. SCHWINDT, "Steps in production of motoneuron spikes during rhythmic firing," *Journal of Neurophysiology* 35:311-325 (1972).

WILLIAM H. CALVIN, JOHN D. LOESER, "Doublet and burst firing patterns within the dorsal column nuclei of cat and man," *Experimental Neurology* 48:406-426 (1975).

WILLIAM H. CALVIN, GEORGE W. SYPERT, "Fast and slow pyramidal tract neurons: An intracellular analysis of their contrasting repetitive firing properties in the cat," *Journal of Neurophysiology* 39:420-434 (1976).

WILLIAM H. CALVIN, DANIEL K. HARTLINE, "Retrograde invasion of lobster stretch receptor somata in the control of firing rate and extra spike patterning," *Journal of Neurophysiology* 40:106-118 (1977).

42 A. J. ROCKEL, R. W. HIORNS, T. P. S. POWELL, "The basic uniformity in structure of the neocortex," *Brain* 103:221-244 (1980). They estimate about 110 neurons in a minicolumn.

43 There is a reason for starting with color: the blobs might help to fix the orientation of the triangular arrays.

43 Binding (see Glossary), e.g., the "temporal tagging" hypothesis of FRANCIS CRICK AND CHRISTOF KOCH, "Some reflections on visual awareness," *Cold Spring Harbor Symposiums in Quantitative Biology* LV:953-962 (1990).

45 Also, let me repeat my caution (p. 36) about perfect regularity: just as the triangular array nodes might be equidistant in travel time rather than distance, so the hexagons need not be perfect in terms of equidistant corresponding points. The possibility that the terminal patches simply self-organize in development, in only roughly triangular fashion, also suggests that the mosaics could look more like Penrose tilings than hexagonal mosaics. This would be particularly likely where cortex is markedly curved, as at the top and bottom of a sulcus (any volleyball will demonstrate how a spherical surface can use hexagons intermixed with pentagons).

45   WILLIAM H. CALVIN, "Error-correcting codes: Coherent hexagonal copying from fuzzy neuroanatomy," *World Congress on Neural Networks* 1:101-104 (1993).

Chapter 4. Managing the Cerebral Commons

51   MICHAEL A. ARBIB, *In Search of the Person* (University of Massachusetts Press 1985), pp.52-53.

52   BARBARA L. FINLAY and RICHARD B. DARLINGTON, "Linked regularities in the development and evolution of mammalian brains," *Science* 268:1578-1584 (16 June 1995).

53   CHARLES DARWIN, *On the Origin of Species* (John Murray, London, 1859, p. 200) notes that "every detail of structure... may be viewed as having been of special use to some ancestral form . . . — either directly, or indirectly through the complex laws of growth."

53   Conversion and coexistence of functions in the same structure: DARWIN (1859), p.137.

53   Language cortex isn't exclusively related to language: see the first few chapters of CALVIN AND OJEMANN (1994).

54   CICERO, *De oratore.*

54   GARRETT HARDIN, "The tragedy of the commons," *Science* 162:1243-1248 (1968).

56   Cartesian theater fallacy, see DANIEL C. DENNETT, *Consciousness Explained* (Little, Brown 1991).

58   For human motor cortex, there is nice evidence that, as one learns a serial reaction time task, the excitability of relevant regions of cortex increases, as seen by wider areas from which a standard transcranial magnetic stimulus could elicit an EMG response from relevant muscle groups. By the time that reaction time finally reaches a maintained minimum, however, the area drops. See ALVARO PASCUAL-LEONE, JORDAN GRAFMAN, MARK HALLETT, "Modulation of cortical motor output maps during development of implicit and explicit knowledge," *Science* 263:1287-1289 (1994). While this expansion might correspond to bigger hexagonal territories, it could also correspond to generating a variety of alternate motor programs, with the final drop corresponding to no longer needing to flounder around.

58   Mass action in the nervous system (also the title of a classic 1975 book by the neurophysiologist Walter J. Freeman) is an old theme in neurophysiology, best presented in Freeman's *Societies of Brains* (Erlbaum 1995).

61 KARL POPPER (1979), quoted by Raphael Sassower in *Cultural Collisions: Postmodern Technoscience* (Routledge).

61 DONALD T. CAMPBELL, "Epistemological roles for selection theory," *Evolution, Cognition, and Realism: Studies in Evolutionary Epistemology, edited by* N. (Lanham, MD: University Press of America 1990), pp. 1-19 at p. 9.

Chapter 5. Resonating with your Chaotic Memories

63 CICERO (104-43 B.C.), *Tusculan Disputions.*

FRIEDRICH WILHELM NIETZSCHE, p. 360 in W. H. Auden and L. Kronenberger, *The Viking Book of Aphorisms* (Viking 1962).

GEORGE SANTAYANA, p. 323 in Auden and Kronenberger (1962).

63 Finches, see WEINER (1994).

64 "Activating the EEG" in small regions of neocortex: ITZHAK FRIED, GEORGE OJEMANN, EBERHARD FETZ, "Language-related potentials specific to human language cortex," *Science* 212:353-356 (1981).

64 ELIZABETH F. LOFTUS, *Eyewitness Testimony* (Harvard University Press 1979).

See SPORNS AND TONINI (1994) and CALVIN AND OJEMANN (1994, chapters 7 and 8) for a summary of the editing of preexisting connections.

66 Chaos, see ABRAHAM et al (1990), FREEMAN (1995), and STEWART (1995).

66 Flutters like a butterfly: FREEMAN (1995), p. 63.

67 The bursting behavior that one sees in epileptic foci of cerebral cortex in between seizures is not necessarily a little seizure: W. H. CALVIN, "Normal repetitive firing and its pathophysiology." In: *Epilepsy: A Window to Brain Mechanisms*, J. Lockard and A. A. Ward, Jr., eds. (Raven Press 1980), pp. 97-121.

For an application of chaos theory to the bursting problem, see STEVEN J. SCHIFF et al, "Controlling chaos in the brain," *Nature* 370:615-620 (1994).

For the role of synchronous input, see X. WANG, M. M. MERZENICH, K. SAMESHIMA, W. M. JENKINS, "Remodeling of hand representation in adult cortex determined by timing of tactile stimulation," *Nature* 378:71-75 (1995).

MARKUS MEISTER, LEON LAGNADO, DENIS A. BAYLOR, "Concerted signaling by retinal ganglion cells," *Science* 270:1207-1210 (17 November 1995).

68 PATRICIA K. KUHL, "Learning and representation in speech and language." *Current Opinion in Neurobiology* 4:812-822 (1994).

69   FREEMAN (1995), p. 67.

70   A discussion of LTP, and of activity-dependent structural changes at synapses, can be found in most neurobiology texts, such as ERIC R. KANDEL, JAMES H. SCHWARTZ, THOMAS M. JESSELL, *Principles of Neural Science*, 3d edition (Elsevier 1991).

70   KARL S. LASHLEY, *Brain Mechanisms and Intelligence* (University of Chicago Press 1929).

71   For some background on the problem of assembling the ensemble, see WOLF SINGER, "Development and plasticity of cortical processing architectures," *Science* 270:758-764 (3 November 1995).

74   PETER A. GETTING, "Emerging principles governing the operation of neural networks," *Annual Reviews of Neuroscience* 12:185-204 (1989).

75   NMDA channel properties, see CHARLES F. STEVENS, "Two principles of brain organization: a challenge for artificial neural networks," in *The Neurobiology of Neural Networks*, edited by Daniel Gardner (MIT Press 1993), pp. 13-20 at p.18.

75   This is perhaps not the time to talk about temporal summation (see the random arrivals examples in CALVIN 1980, cited later) but it should be noted that NMDA channels also contribute to a slower decay of EPSPs and thus greater summation for an additional reason. Furthermore, the calcium ion entry through an NMDA channel likely stimulates various second messenger mechanisms inside the neuron.

76   Information is just becoming available for the layer 5 pyramidal neurons from loose patch recordings on both soma and apical dendrite. Action potentials consistently following EPSPs may enhance them by 20 percent but it takes fairly large voltage changes, perhaps even calcium spikes nearby, to effectively condition the EPSPs. See GREG STUART AND BERT SAKMANN, "Amplification of EPSPs by axosomatic sodium channels in neocortical pyramidal neurons," *Neuron* 15:1065-1076 (1995).

A. M. BROWN, PETER C. SCHWINDT, WAYNE CRILL, "Different voltage dependence of transient and persistent Na^+ currents is compatible with modal-gating hypothesis for sodium channels," *Journal of Neurophysiology* 71:2562-2565 (1994).

77   One simple theory is that there are two calcium-current thresholds in dendrites, the lower one associated with long-term depression and the higher one with long-term potentiation. See C. HANSEL, A. ARTOLA, WOLF SINGER, "Ca^{2+} signals associated with the induction of long-term potentiation and long-term depression in pyramidal cells of the rat visual cortex," *Society for Neuroscience Abstracts* 711.3 (1995).

77   Cortical neurons are individually capable of firing rhythmically to sustained inputs: WILLIAM H. CALVIN, GEORGE W. SYPERT, "Fast and slow pyramidal tract neurons: An intracellular analysis of their contrasting repetitive firing properties in the cat," *Journal of Neurophysiology* 39:420-434 (1976).

77 W. R. SOFTKY, CHRISTOF KOCH, "The highly irregular firing of cortical cells is inconsistent with temporal integration of random EPSPs," *Journal of Neuroscience* 13:334-50 (1993).

77 *Mea culpa.* I spent a fair amount of time trying to convince people that cortical neurons ought to fire rhythmically, just like motor neurons, that they were impressively *analog*: W. H. CALVIN, "Normal repetitive firing and its pathophysiology," in *Epilepsy: A Window to Brain Mechanisms* (J. Lockard and A. A. Ward, Jr., eds.), Raven Press, New York, pp. 97-121 (1980). The analog aspects may, of course, still be a major factor in the dendritic amplification of synaptic inputs, even in those cases where coincidence detection seems to be the name of the game: see *Coincidence Detection in the Nervous System*, edited by JENNIFER ALTMAN (Human Frontier Science Program, Strasbourg 1996).

78 Lots of triangular array activity would be my favorite candidate for a region of neocortex doing something interesting, not overall levels of activity as indicated by blood flow or metabolism. Note that, in the transition from disorganized activity to sharpened-up triangular arrays, an AGC might effectively mask such more traditional indicators of neocortical "activity." More firing would occur at nodes of triangular arrays, and less would occur nearby, thanks to the AGC — and there might be no net change in the activity spatially averaged for a blood-flow-based technique to detect.

79 ABELES (1991).

79 PETER KÖNIG, ANDRAS K. ENGEL, WOLF SINGER, "Relation between oscillatory activity and long-range synchronization in cat visual cortex," *Proceedings of the National Academy of Sciences U.S.A.* 92:290-294 (1995).

79 HERBERT A. SIMON, *The Sciences of the Artificial* (MIT Press 1969), pp. 95-96.

Chapter 6. Partitioning the Playfield

81 JOHN Z. YOUNG, *A Model of the Brain* (Claredon Press 1964). His "The organization of a memory system," *Proceedings of the Royal Society* (London) 163B:285-320 (1965) introduces the mnemon concept in which weakened synapses serve to tune up a function. A later version is his "Learning as a process of selection," *Journal of the Royal Society of Medicine* 72:801-804 (1979).

81 RICHARD DAWKINS, "Selective neurone death as a possible memory mechanism," *Nature* 229:118-119 (1971).

82   JEAN-PIERRE CHANGEUX, A. DANCHIN, "Selective stabilization of developing synapses as a mechanism for the specification of neuronal networks," *Nature* 264:705-712 (1976).

82   GERALD M. EDELMAN, "Group selection and phasic reentrant signaling: a theory of higher brain function," in *The Neurosciences Fourth Study Program*, edited by F. O. Schmitt and F. G. Worden, pp. 1115-1139 (MIT Press 1979).

82   Three-fold range in size of primary visual cortex among adults: SUZANNE S. STENSAAS, D. K. EDDINGTON, AND W. H. DOBELLE, "The topography and variability of the primary visual cortex in man," *Journal of Neurosurgery* 40:747-755 (June 1974).

82   For a recent version of the silent synapse story, see PATRICK D. WALL, "Do nerve impulses penetrate terminal arborizations? A pre-presynaptic control mechanism," *Trends in Neurosciences* 18:99-103 (February 1995).

82   OTTO RÖSSLER, "The chaotic hierarchy," *Zeitschrift für Natur-forschung* 38A:788-802 (1983).

82   GERALD M. EDELMAN, *Neural Darwinism* (Basic Books 1987).

WILLIAM H. CALVIN, "A global brain theory (a book review of Gerald Edelman's *Neural Darwinism*)," *Science* 240:1802-1803 (24 June 1988).

83   "Differential amplification of particular variants in a population," is from EDELMAN (1989), p. 39.

83   "[This] is a population theory," EDELMAN (1987), p. 31.

85   Overwriting: LOFTUS (1979).

85   Hippocampus does replay firing sequences during sleep: see WILLIAM E. SKAGGS, BRUCE L. MACNAUGHTON, "Replay of neuronal firing sequences in rat hippocampus during sleep following spatial experience," *Science* 271:1870-1873 (29 March 1996).

85   G. BUZHÁKI, A. BRAGIN, J. J. CHROBAK, Z. NÁDASDY, A. SIK, M. HSU, A. YLINEN, "Oscillatory and intermittent synchrony in the hippocampus: relevance to memory trace formation," pp. 145-172. in *Temporal Coding in the Brain*, edited by G. BUZHÁKI et al (Springer 1994).

85   "Timing jitter" is also easily solved via lots of clones. The modern version of the "throwing theory" is in WILLIAM H. CALVIN, "The unitary hypothesis: A common neural circuitry for novel manipulations, language, plan-ahead, and throwing?" pp. 230-250 in *Tools, Language, and Cognition in Human Evolution*, edited by Kathleen R. Gibson and Tim Ingold (Cambridge University Press 1993).

86   Hyperacuity in sensation: WILLIAM H. CALVIN, "Precision timing requirements suggest wider brain connections, not more restricted ones," *Behavioral and Brain Sciences* 7:334 (1984).

86   Evolutionarily stable strategies (ESSs), see JOHN MAYNARD SMITH, *The Evolution of Sex* (Cambridge University Press 1978).

88   Actually, because axons may have several clusters of terminals along a run, spaced "0.5 mm" apart, gateways do not have to be open, only thin.

95   Niche quote is from ERNST MAYR, *Toward a New Philosophy of Biology* (Harvard University Press 1988), p. 135. In G. E. Hutchinson's definition, niche is a multidimensional resource space.

95   Borneo quote is from MAYR (1988), p. 136.

96   Potential niche space: MAYR (1988), p. 129.

96   Spreadsheet evolution is discussed in my book, *The River that Flows Uphill* (Sierra Club Books 1987), Day 13.

97   Evolutionarily stable strategies (ESSs) surely constitute a meta-level for the cortical competitions. Just as they explained why immediate self-interest wasn't always the name of the game for the prisoner's dilemma and the like, so ESSs will probably prove relevant to the work space competitions. Once simulation of a neocortical Darwin machine handles the simple competitions, it will be interesting to see what cooperative phenomena are like. But it lies beyond the capabilities of the present analysis, that primarily relies on the mosaics of plane geometry for explanatory power.

98   JAMES L. GOULD and CAROL GRANT GOULD, *The Animal Mind*, Scientific American Library, p. 43, 1994.

WILLIAM JAMES, "Great men, great thoughts, and the environment," *The Atlantic Monthly* 46(276):441-459 (October 1880).

Intermission Notes

The chalk drawing of Charles Darwin in the 1840s is by Samuel Laurence. A color reproduction can be seen on the dust jacket of JANET BROWNE's *Charles Darwin, Volume 1, Voyaging* (1995). The original is at Darwin's country home, Down House, in the London suburbs (directions: *http://weber.u.washington.edu/~wcalvin/down_hse.html*).

104   ROY M. PRITCHARD, WOODBURN HERON, DONALD O. HEBB, "Visual perception approached by the method of stabilized images," *Canadian Journal of Psychology* 14:67-77 (1960).

The subject's profile, adapted from HEBB (1980, the source of the history), was redrawn from a photograph appearing in ROY M. PRITCHARD, "Stabilized images on the retina," *Scientific American* 204:72-78 (June 1961).

105 The Cheshire Cat makes its (dis)appearance in LEWIS CARROLL, *Alice's Adventures in Wonderland* (1865).

106 Sustained firing can occur from sustained inputs or from a bias in leakage currents that creates a pacemaker: see, for example, WILLIAM H. CALVIN, CHARLES F. STEVENS, "Synaptic noise and other sources of randomness in motoneuron interspike intervals," *Journal of Neurophysiology* 31:574-587 (1968).

106 For an appreciation of Hebb by his former student and long-time colleague, PETER M. MILNER (who also helped extend Hebb's cell-assembly to categories and to synchrony), see "The mind and Donald O. Hebb," *Scientific American* 268(1):124-129 (January 1993), and "Neural representations: some old problems revisited," *Journal of Cognitive Neuroscience* 8:69-77 (January 1996).

106 Hebb introduced all three major concepts for which he is now celebrated — first the dual trace memory, then the cell-assembly, and finally the Hebbian synapse — in just two consecutive pages (pp. 61-62) of *The Organization of Behavior.* In many places in the book, he is most apologetic and defensive about burdening readers with his speculations — but Hebb, in addition to the physiological orientation he received as a student of Karl Lashley's, had an overriding conviction that theory was worth doing. This conviction was seldom shared by neuroscientists of his day, who were thoroughly impatient with theory. The situation was nothing like the healthy competition between experimentalists and theoreticians that has long existed in physics. Indeed, in the midst of my two decades of experimental work when I started doing theory part-time, theory was much maligned and there were only several full-time theorists working in neuroscience-like departments. It was only when connectionism caught everyone's attention in the mid-1980s that doing theory finally became halfway respectable among neuroscientists. And one of the things that everyone was then talking about were those retrogradely-strengthened synapses, predicted four decades earlier amidst much apology by Hebb.

107 RICHARD DAWKINS, "Viruses of the mind," in *Dennett and His Critics: Demystifying Mind,* edited by Bo Dahlbom (Blackwell 1993). And see RICHARD BRODIE, *Virus of the Mind* (Integral Press, Seattle 1995).

108 Permission to memorize: FRANKLIN B. KRASNE, "Extrinsic control of intrinsic neuronal plasticity: a hypothesis from work on simple systems," *Brain Research* 140:197-206 (1978).

111 J. ALLAN HOBSON, *The Chemistry of Conscious States* (Little, Brown 1994), p.117.

111 HEBB (1980), p. 5.

Chapter 7. The Brownian Notion

113 IMMANUEL KANT, *Critique of Pure Reason* (1781; translation St. Martins Press 1965), p. A141.

114 Eleanor Rosch, see JOHNSON (1987).

114 SAMUEL BUTLER ("II"), quoted at p. 333 by W. H. Auden and L. Kronenberger, *The Viking Book of Aphorisms* (Viking 1962).

114 BICKERTON (1995), pp. 51-52.

116 Simple associative memories: see DANIEL L. ALKON, *Memory's Voice* (HarperCollins 1992).

119 ROBERT HOLT, "The microevolutionary consequences of climate change," *Trends in Evolution and Ecology* 5:311-315 (1990).

120 FREEMAN (1995), p. 100.

121 "Future place cells," see L. F. ABBOTT, K. I. BLUM, "Learning and generating motor sequences," *Nervous Systems and Behaviour* (Proceedings of the 4th International Congress of Neuroethology), p.106 (1995).

121 Efference copy dates back to E. VON HOLST, H. MITTELSTAEDT, "Das Reafferenzprinzip. Wechselwiskungen zwischen Zentralnervensystem und Peripherie," *Naturwissenschaften* 37:464-476 (1950).

122 J. ALLAN HOBSON, *The Chemistry of Conscious States* (Little, Brown 1994), pp. 59-60.

123 "Titles to abstracts to full texts" is going to be extended, thanks to web pages where five-minute audio-visual presentations can be added. And even the half-hour canned lab tour, for the very curious, with options that demonstrate lab techniques.

123 BRUCE SCHNEIER, *Applied Cryptography* (Wiley 1994), p.28.

125 My musical history is taken from that of STEVEN R. HOLTZMAN, *Digital Mantras: The Languages of Abstract and Virtual Worlds* (MIT Press 1994), pp. 18-33.

126 Particularly relevant among the cortical theories is KRISHNA V. SHENOY, JEFFREY KAUFMAN, JOHN V. MCGRANN, GORDON L. SHAW, "Learning by selection in the trion model of cortical organization," *Cerebral Cortex* 3:239-248 (1993).

127 HEBB (1980), p. 107.

Chapter 8. Convergence Zones and a Hint of Sex

129 JOHN MAYNARD SMITH, *The Theory of Evolution* (Cambridge University Press 1993), p. 41.

130 Conduction speed in axons is a function of their diameter, the extent of their myelin wrapping, and the density of sodium channels at their nodes of Ranvier. Because sodium channels are regularly replaced, up-regulating the insertion of new channels could easily be used to increase conduction speed on a side branch. Minor hesitations at branch points also enter into consideration, though the synaptic delay is the largest hesitation — and the most easily varied, if tuning to equalize travel time. For a theoretical analysis, see Y. MANOR, CHRISTOF KOCH, IDAN SEGEV, "Effect of geometrical irregularities on propagation delay in axonal trees," *Biophysical Journal* 60:1424-1437 (1991).

131 I thank my colleague JOHN W. SUNSTEN for the whole brain photographs; they are among the excellent collection at *http://www1.biostr.-washington.edu/DigitalAnatomist.html*.

131 Mapping corticocorticals with strychnine: J. G. DUSSER DE BARENNE, W. S. MCCULLOCH, "Functional organization of the sensory cortex of the monkey," *Journal of Neurophysiology* 1:69-85 (1938).

131 For the columns and layers summary, see WILLIAM H. CALVIN, "Cortical columns, modules, and Hebbian cell assemblies," in *Handbook of Brain Theory and Neural Networks*, M. A. ARBIB, ed. (MIT Press 1995), pp. 269-272.

131 Convergence zones, see ANTONIO R. DAMASIO, "Time-locked multiregional retroactivation: a systems-level proposal for the neural substrates of recall and recognition," *Cognition* 33:25-62 (1989). For a good example of corticocortical connectivity, see TERRY W. DEACON, "Cortical connections of the inferior arcuate sulcus cortex in the macaque brain," *Brain Research* 573:8-26 (1992).

132 Detail of PABLO PICASSO, *Woman in an Armchair* (1941), Musée Picasso, Paris.

134 Temporal summation of inputs, see pp. 105 of CALVIN AND OJEMANN (1994).

134 Time window of NMDA channel (at room temperature): J. M. BEKKERS, C. F. STEVENS, "Computational implications of NMDA receptor channels," *Cold Spring Harbor Symposia on Quantitative Biology* LV:131-135 (1990).

136 Another contributor to submerging the less successful is long-term depression (LTD), a reduction in synaptic strengths that occurs with conditioning stimuli that are insufficient to evoke long-term potentiation (LTP). While it is still unclear whether LTD is actually a synaptic mechanism or a reduction in dendritic amplification by calcium and sodium currents, it should have the desirable feature of reducing the size of the hot spot.

137 Gamete dimorphism, see LYNN MARGULIS and DORION SAGAN (Yale University Press 1986) and MAYNARD SMITH (1978).

138 Setup for sexual selection to operate: for a more complete discussion, see CRONIN (1991), p.114.

140 I say "loosely analogous" because the sperm-ova dimorphism isn't due to small vs. large quantities of DNA but rather of stored energy. Still, ova *do* have somewhat more DNA because of the maternal-only mitochondrial mtDNA and the female's two X chromosomes.

141 Synesthesia is described in RICHARD E. CYTOWIC, *The Man Who Tasted Shapes* (Putnams 1993).

144 HENRY J. PERKINSON, *Teachers Without Goals/Students Without Purposes* (McGraw-Hill 1993), p. 34.

DAMIEN BRODERICK (1996). See *http://odyssey.apana.org.au/~terminus/iq-14.html#Interview with Damien Broderick*

Chapter 9. Chimes on the Quarter Hour

145 ROGER SHANK and ROBERT ABELSON, *Scripts, Plans, Goals and Understanding* (Erlbaum 1977), p. 41.

Urge to finish known sequence serving to quiet crying children: SANDRA TREHUB, University of Toronto, personal communication (1995).

PETER BROOKS, *Reading for the Plot: Design and Intention in Narrative* (Random House 1984), pp. 1-2.

146 *Jabberwocky* later appeared in LEWIS CARROLL, *Through the Looking Glass*.

147 DENNETT (1995), p.139.

147 Hint: the next line is "The evil that men do lives after them. . . ." The answer is in the notes for the last chapter.

150 GORDON H. BOWER and DANIEL G. MORROW, "Mental models in narrative comprehension," *Science* 247:44-48 (1990).

151 J. HORE, S. WATTS, J. MARTIN, B. MILLER. "Timing of finger opening and ball release in fast and accurate overarm throws," *Experimental Brain Research* 103: 277-286 (1995).

J. HORE, S. WATTS, D. TWEED, "Arm position constraints when throwing in three dimensions," *Journal of Neurophysiology* 72: 1171-1180 (1994).

151 WILLIAM H. CALVIN, CHARLES F. STEVENS, "Synaptic noise as a source of variability in the interval between action potentials," *Science* 155:842-844 (1967).

152   WILLIAM H. CALVIN, "A stone's throw and its launch window: timing precision and its implications for language and hominid brains," *Journal of Theoretical Biology* 104:121-135 (1983).

152   WILLIAM H. CALVIN, GEORGE W. SYPERT, "Fast and slow pyramidal tract neurons: An intracellular analysis of their contrasting repetitive firing properties in the cat," *Journal of Neurophysiology* 39:420-434 (1976).

153   JOHN R. CLAY, ROBERT DEHAAN, "Fluctuations in interbeat interval in rhythmic heart-cell clusters," *Biophysical Journal* 28:377-389 (1979).

153   J. T. ENRIGHT, "Temporal precision in circadian systems: a reliable neuronal clock from unreliable components?" *Science* 209:1542-1544 (1980).

154   BRIAN ENO, radio interview on *Fresh Air* (1990) and personal communication (1995).

154   See my mention of NMDA effects in chapter 7. There my example was correcting offcourse arm trajectories, but it equally applies to subvocal sequences.

155   A good physiologically oriented book on music is by the neurologist FRANK R. WILSON, *Tone Deaf and All Thumbs?* (Viking Penguin 1986). The illustration showing the bifurcating path of a pendulum attracted by several magnets was made using *James Gleick's CHAOS: The Software* (Autodesk 1991).

157   JOHN HOLLAND, "Complex adaptive systems," *Daedalus* (Winter 1992), p. 25.

Chapter 10. The Making of Metaphor

159   SAMUEL P. HUNTINGTON, "If not civilizations, what?" *Foreign Affairs* 72(5):186-194 (1993).

159   MICHAEL REDDY, "The conduit metaphor," in A. Ortony (ed.), *Metaphor and Thought* (Cambridge University Press 1979).

159   The art of the good guess is discussed by CALVIN (1996).

159   ALLAN SANDAGE, quoted by Timothy Ferris in *The New Yorker*, p. 50 (15 May 1995).

160   "Without imagination...": HAROLD OSBORNE, *Aesthetics and Art Theory* (Dutton 1970), p.208.

161   FREEMAN (1995), p. 107.

161   Schema is used for knowledge structures in general, but I am using it in JOHNSON'S (1987, p.2) sense of an image schema, a dynamic pattern that functions somewhat like an abstract version of an image, thereby connecting up a vast range of different experiences that manifest similar properties.

161 My grammar exposition derives from that of Derek Bickerton, *Language and Species* (University of Chicago Press 1990). In human language cortex, the layer 3 pyramidal neurons are consistently larger in the left hemisphere: J. J. Hutsler, M. S. Gazzaniga, "Acetylcholinesterase staining in human auditory and language cortices: regional variation of structural features," *Cerebral Cortex* 6:260-270 (April 1996).

161 Containment, see Johnson (1987), p.126.

162 P. Iverson, Patricia K. Kuhl, "Mapping the perceptual magnet effect for speech using signal detection theory and multidimensional scaling," *Journal of the Acoustical Society of America* 97:553-562 (1995).

163 Nancy J. C. Andreasen, Pauline S. Powers, "Creativity and psychosis: An examination of conceptual style," *Archives of General Psychiatry* 32:70-73 (1975).

164 Dedre Genter, Donald Genter, "Flowing water or teeming crowds: mental models of electricity," in Dedre Genter and Albert Stevens (eds.), *Mental Models* (Erlbaum 1983), pp.99-129.

164 Hans Selye, see Johnson (1987), chapter 5.

165 Marvin Minsky, *The Society of Mind* (Simon & Schuster 1987), ch. 20.

166 "One then reduces the excitability until only the better resonances remain active." This is not unlike reducing the temperature in the DNA annealing technique, judging the percentage of zipped-up DNA fragments from the temperature at which the solution's surface first coalesces.

166 Henry Moore, quoted at p.26 by Ken Macrorie, *Telling Writing*, 3d ed. (Hayden Book Company 1980).

167 Note that if a spatiotemporal pattern did not need to be spatially cloned, in order to gain the attention of output pathways, the spatial extent of attractors could be less than a hexagon pair. But that would give a lot of power to very few cells, and a chorus requirement would be safer.

169 I have discussed the common neural machinery for speech and hand movements most recently in William H. Calvin, "The unitary hypothesis: A common neural circuitry for novel manipulations, language, plan-ahead, and throwing?" pp. 230-250 in *Tools, Language, and Cognition in Human Evolution*, edited by Kathleen R. Gibson and Tim Ingold (Cambridge University Press 1993).

169 "Vice versa...." Calvin (1993).

170 George A. Ojemann, "Brain organization for language from the perspective of electrical stimulation mapping," *Behavioral and Brain Sciences* 6(2):189-230 (June 1983).

170 Bickerton (1990), p.86.

236

170 JACOB BRONOWSKI, *The Origins of Knowledge and Imagination* (Yale University Press 1978, transcribed from 1967 lectures).
171 KENNETH J. W. CRAIK, *The Nature of Explanation* (Cambridge University Press 1943).
172 Narrative unity: see, for example, PAUL RICOEUR, *Time and Narrative* (University of Chicago Press 1984).
172 HEINZ PAGELS, *The Dreams of Reason* (Simon & Schuster 1988).

Chapter 11. Thinking a Thought in the Mosaics of the Mind

175 DANIEL C. DENNETT, *Darwin's Dangerous Idea* (Simon & Schuster 1995), p. 460. And, since I did promise you the answer to Dennett's puzzler, X is:

```
Pdun Dqwrqb'v idprxv ixqhudo rudwlrq lq Zlooldp
Vkdnhvshduh'v Mxolxv Fdhvdu, Dfw LLL Vfhqh 2:
"Iulhqgv, Urpdqv, frxqwubphq, ohqg ph brxu hduv;
L frph wr exub Fdhvdu, qrw wr sudlvh klp."
```

Well, to keep you from involuntarily seeing the answer, I've encrypted it with the famous Caesar Cipher where each plaintext character is replaced by the one located three to the right in modulo 26. I've left the number and the punctuation unencrypted.

```
ABCDEFGHIJKLMNOPQRSTUVWXYZ plaintext
DEFGHIJKLMNOPQRSTUVWXYZABC ciphertext
```

176 KARL R. POPPER AND JOHN C. ECCLES, *The Self and Its Brain* (Springer 1977)
176 EUGEN HERRIGEL, *Zen in the Art of Archery* (Pantheon 1953).
180 JONATHAN WEINER, *The Beak of the Finch* (Knopf 1994), p. 129.
181 J. B. S. HALDANE, *Journal of Genetics* 58 (1963).
181 For a history of the confusions about levels of explanation and mechanism, see HELENA CRONIN, *The Ant and the Peacock* (1991).
181 Ignorance of levels of explanation: see my *How Brains Think*, chapter three, "The janitor's dream."
181 WILLIAM JAMES, *Principles of Psychology* (1890).
182 FRANCIS CRICK and CHRISTOF KOCH, ``The problem of consciousness,'' *Scientific American* 267(3):152-159 (September 1992). The Neural Correlate of Consciousness (their NCC) is some relevant group of neurons firing in some relevant pattern for a sufficient duration. It is easy to imagine how population-style hegemony could be their NCC, but I would caution that passive awareness may be much simpler than the creative constructs implied by the James-Piaget-Popper levels of

consciousness; a pop-through recognition of a familiar object may not need to utilize a cloning competition in the manner of an ambiguous percept or a novel movement.

183 EDELMAN (1989), p. 148.

183 PAUL VALÉRY, quoted at p. 346 in W. H. Auden and L. Kronenberger, *The Viking Book of Aphorisms* (Viking 1962).

183 Dreaming: HOBSON (1988).

185 "Too slow." One of our best ways of compensating for insufficient amounts of neurotransmitters is to increase the time it dwells in the synaptic cleft. But drugs that delay transmitter breakdown or sequestration thereby change the time constants, and so slow the natural fluctuations.

186 KAY REDFIELD JAMISON, *An Unquiet Mind: A Memoir of Moods and Madness* (Knopf 1995).

186 Mixed depression: FREDERICK K. GOODWIN, KAY REDFIELD JAMISON, *Manic-depressive Illness* (Oxford University Press 1990), p.48.

187 HOBSON (1994).

187 HEBB (1980), p. 26.

188 Joan of Arc: CALVIN & OJEMANN (1994), p. 79.

188 "Some long-ago success" might, at one extreme, be the tuning-up period of ontogeny when diffuse wiring is pruned, leaving only those terminal clusters that have been engaging in a test pattern.

189 Functional roles for EEG rhythms: discussed by THEODORE H. BULLOCK,"How do brains work?" chapter 10 in *Induced rhythms in the brain*, edited by E. Basar, T. H. Bullock (Birkhauser 1991).

189 WALLACE STEVENS, from "Adagia," in *Opus Posthumous* (Knopf 1957).

191 Our modern experience with packet data transmission illustrates one way that a serial-order bottleneck can be circumvented, allowing the same channel to be simultaneously used for several tasks (internet telephony, text file transfer, and image download, all going over the same twisted pair wire). Frequency multiplexing is another, as is time slicing. So until we have pushed the issue hard enough with experimental techniques, it may be well to remember that the "unity of consciousness" is not the settled issue that it first appears.

191 Attractors that fade more slowly might still fade out overnight, provided that sleep processes protected the cortical area from writing new ones. REM sleep process do, after all, inhibit many muscles; also inhibiting the cortical areas used for agendas might function much like the mantras of my *Intermission Notes*.

192 GEORGE STEINER, "Has truth a future?" Bronowski memorial lecture, reprinted in Bernard Dixon, editor, *From Creation to Chaos* (Basil

Blackwell 1989), pp. 234-252 at p.250. Simply "being interested in something," as Steiner likes to say, is a form of evolving agenda that structures the daily lives of creative people. There are likely multiple evolving agendas in no particular hierarchy, as when one interrupts writing the magnum opus to do the laundry — and then again, an hour later, when one remembers to water the dehydrated house plants.

194 BICKERTON (1990). For some of the elements needed for a Universal Grammar, see JACKENDOFF (1993), p. 81, pp. 159-164; BICKERTON (1995), pp.30ff; and NOAM CHOMSKY, "A minimalist program for linguistic theory," pp. 1-52 in *The View from Building 20* (MIT Press 1993), edited by K. Hale and S. J. Keyser (it's a WW2 "temporary building" at M.I.T.; back in 1961-62, I had an office in 20B-225). It is thought that a mechanism for recursive embedding buys you the most important aspects of UG.

196 WILLIAM H. CALVIN, "The emergence of Universal Grammar from protolanguage: corticocortical coherence could enable binding and recursive embedding," *Society for Neuroscience Abstracts* 22 (1996).

199 DARWIN (1859).

Glossary and Brief Tutorials

203 See STEWART (1995), p.117.

204 For more on chaos, start with chapter 8 of STEWART (1995) before progressing to ABRAHAM (1990), GLASS AND MACKEY (1990), and FREEMAN (1995).

206 Discussions of unitary processes can be found in WILLIAM H. CALVIN and KATHERINE GRAUBARD, "Styles of neuronal computation," chapter 29 in *The Neurosciences, Fourth Study Program*, edited by F. O. Schmitt and F. G. Worden (MIT Press 1979).

206 HELENA CRONIN, *The Ant and the Peacock* (Cambridge University Press 1991), p.107.

206 Genetic code: see any biology text or DOUGLAS HOFSTADTER *Metamagical Themas* (BasicBooks 1985), pp.672ff.

212 Resonance: see, for example, STEWART (1995), pp. 24-25.

The Author

After an early flirtation with photojournalism and electrical engineering, I majored in physics at Northwestern University (B.A., 1961), spent a year at M.I.T. and Harvard Medical School absorbing the atmosphere of what eventually became known as neuroscience, then went to the University of Washington to do a degree in physiology and biophysics (Ph.D., 1966) working under Charles F. Stevens. I subsequently stayed in Seattle, spending 20 years on the faculty of the Department of Neurological Surgery at the other end of the building, a wonderful postdoctoral education as 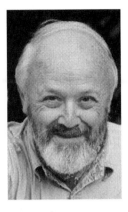 well as a home for my theoretical and experimental work on neuron repetitive firing mechanisms. After a 1978–79 sabbatical as visiting professor of neurobiology at the Hebrew University of Jerusalem, my interests began to shift toward theoretical issues in the ensemble properties of neural circuits — and to the big brain problem of hominid evolution. Friends in psychology, zoology, archaeology, and physical anthropology tried hard to educate me as I stumbled into their fields during the 1980s. As I began writing books and royalty advances arrived, I increasingly took unpaid leave, stopped writing grant applications, and shed responsibilities. Other university researchers may spend a third of their time teaching students and coping with the bureaucracy; I now spend about the same proportion of my time writing books for general readers and coping with publishers. For some years now, I have been an affiliate member of the faculty of the Department of Psychiatry and Behavioral Sciences at the University of Washington — again a wonderful education, though I am no more a psychiatrist now than I was a neurosurgeon before. Pressed for a specialization, I usually say that I'm a theoretical neurophysiologist.

Details can be found via my web pages, such as the full text of many of my articles and chapters from each of my books. The links start at *http://weber.u.washington.edu/~wcalvin/*.

240

About the Artists

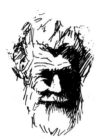

MALCOLM WELLS, who did most of the freehand sketches that are inset into the text, is, among many other things, an architect, author of *Underground Buildings*, the illustrator of my book *How the Shaman Stole the Moon*, and a proprietor of the Underground Art Gallery in Brewster, Massachusetts, out on the biceps of Cape Cod.

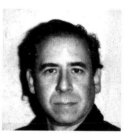

MARK MEYER, who did the cover art, is also a neurobiologist in the Department of Zoology at the University of Washington. Other examples of his art, and guides to his recent paintings, can be found at his web page: *http://weber.u.washington.edu/~mrmeyer*.

Index

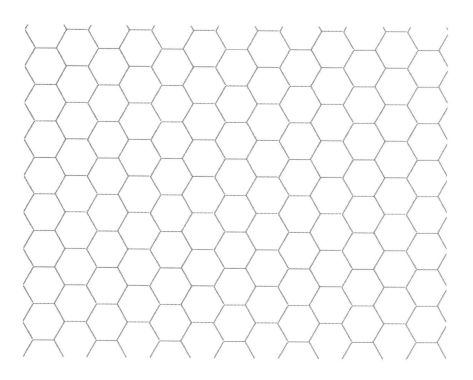

A workspace template